LITTLE,
BROWN

LB

**LARGE
PRINT**

ALSO BY ANDREW WEIL, MD

Fast Food, Good Food: More Than 150 Quick and Easy Ways to Put Healthy, Delicious Food on the Table

True Food: Seasonal, Sustainable, Simple, Pure
(with Sam Fox and Michael Stebner)

Spontaneous Happiness: A New Path to Emotional Well-Being

You Can't Afford to Get Sick: Your Guide to Optimum Health and Health Care
(originally published as *Why Our Health Matters*)

Integrative Oncology (with Donald Abrams, MD)

Healthy Aging: A Lifelong Guide to Your Physical and Spiritual Well-Being

The Healthy Kitchen: Recipes for a Better Body, Life, and Spirit
(with Rosie Daley)

Eating Well for Optimum Health: The Essential Guide to Bringing Health and Pleasure Back to Eating

Eight Weeks to Optimum Health: A Proven Program for Taking Full Advantage of Your Body's Natural Healing Power

Spontaneous Healing: How to Discover and Enhance Your Body's Natural Ability to Maintain and Heal Itself

Natural Health, Natural Medicine: The Complete Guide to Wellness and Self-Care for Optimum Health

Health and Healing: The Philosophy of Integrative Medicine and Optimum Health

From Chocolate to Morphine: Everything You Need to Know About Mind-Altering Drugs (with Winifred Rosen)

The Marriage of the Sun and Moon: Dispatches from the Frontiers of Consciousness

The Natural Mind: A Revolutionary Approach to the Drug Problem

MIND
OVER
MEDS

Know When Drugs Are Necessary,
When Alternatives Are Better—
and When to Let Your Body Heal on Its Own

ANDREW WEIL, MD

LITTLE, BROWN AND COMPANY

LARGE PRINT EDITION

Little, Brown and Company
Hachette Book Group
1290 Avenue of the Americas, New York, NY 10104
littlebrown.com

First Edition: April 2017

Little, Brown and Company is a division of Hachette Book Group, Inc. The Little, Brown name and logo are trademarks of Hachette Book Group, Inc.

The publisher is not responsible for websites (or their content) that are not owned by the publisher.

ISBN 978-0-316-35297-0 (hardcover) / 978-0-316-55241-7 (large print)
LCCN 2016950776

10 9 8 7 6 5 4 3 2 1

LSC-C

Printed in the United States of America

For my colleagues in integrative medicine

Contents

Contents

List of Contributors

The opinions expressed in this book are mine and mine alone. The colleagues listed below supplied information and research data that I used in writing about the various classes of medications discussed in these pages.

CHAPTER 1. ANTIBIOTICS

Maya Shetreat-Klein, MD, is an adult and pediatric neurologist, herbalist, naturalist, and urban farmer in New York City. She is founder and director of the Terrain Institute, a training program in terrain medicine, which explores the relationship between the body and the world around us. She is the author of *The Dirt Cure: Growing Healthy Kids with Food Straight from Soil* (dirtcure.com).

CHAPTER 2. STATINS

Stephen Devries, MD, FACC, is a preventive cardiologist and executive director of the Gaples Institute for Integrative Cardiology outside Chicago, an educational nonprofit organization dedicated to advancing the role of nutrition and lifestyle in health care. Dr. Devries is the coauthor of *What Your Doctor May Not Tell You About Cholesterol* and coeditor of *Integrative Cardiology.*

CHAPTER 3. MEDICATIONS FOR GERD

Gerard Mullin, MD (thefoodmd.com), is associate professor of medicine at the Johns Hopkins Hospital. He has more than twenty years of clinical experience in the field of integrative gastroenterology. His latest book is *The Gut Balance Revolution: Boost Your Metabolism, Restore Your Inner Ecology, and Lose the Weight for Good!*

Alyssa Parian, MD, is assistant professor of medicine at the Johns Hopkins Hospital. She is board certified in internal medicine and gastroenterology and specializes in the treatment of inflammatory bowel disease.

Chapter 4. Antihistamines

Randy Horwitz, MD, PhD, is an internist/allergist/immunologist and associate professor of medicine at the University of Arizona. He also serves as medical director of the University of Arizona Center for Integrative Medicine. He is the coeditor of *Integrative Rheumatology* and the author of the forthcoming book *Integrative Allergy and Asthma*.

Chapter 5. Medications for the Common Cold and the Flu

Russell H. Greenfield, MD, is clinical professor of medicine at the University of North Carolina at Chapel Hill School of Medicine. He maintains an integrative medicine practice in Charlotte and consults with organizations on integrative wellness initiatives.

Chapter 6. Sleep Aids

Rubin Naiman, PhD (DrNaiman.com), is a psychologist, sleep and dream specialist, and clinical assistant professor of medicine at the University of Arizona Center for Integrative Medicine. He is also director of

Circadian Health Associates, an organization that provides training and consultations regarding sleep disorders. Dr. Naiman is the author of a number of books, including *Healing Night*.

CHAPTER 7. STEROIDS

Nisha Manek, MD, is fellowship trained in rheumatology and integrative medicine. She practices integrative rheumatology at HonorHealth Scottsdale Shea Medical Center and at Kingman Regional Medical Center, both in Arizona.

CHAPTER 8. NONSTEROIDAL ANTI-INFLAMMATORY DRUGS (NSAIDs)

Leila Ali-Akbarian, MD-MPH, is a family medicine physician and medical director of the University of Arizona Cancer Center Supportive Care Clinic, where she sees patients in a multi-disciplinary, integrative, supportive-care setting.

Patricia Lebensohn, MD, is a family medicine physician and director of the Integrative Medicine in Residency (IMR) program at the University of Arizona Center for Integrative Medicine. IMR has been adopted by more than sixty residency programs throughout the United States, Taiwan, and Germany.

Mari Ricker, MD, is a family medicine physician and associate director of the Integrative Medicine in Residency Program at the University of Arizona Center for Integrative Medicine.

CHAPTER 9. PSYCHIATRIC MEDICATIONS FOR ADULTS

Jingduan Yang, MD, FAPA (jdyangmd.com), is a psychiatrist, clinical assistant professor of psychiatry, and director of the Acupuncture and Oriental Medicine Program at Thomas Jefferson University Hospital in Philadelphia. He also serves on the teaching faculty of the University of Arizona Center for Integrative Medicine. Dr. Yang is the founder of the Tao Institute of Modern Wellness (taoinstitute .com) and author of the popular book *Facing East: Ancient Health and Beauty Secrets for the Modern Age*.

CHAPTER 11. MEDICATIONS FOR ATTENTION DEFICIT HYPERACTIVITY DISORDER (ADHD)

Sanford Newmark, MD, is a pediatrician and director of clinical programs at the Osher Center for Integrative Medicine at the University of California, San Francisco, where he is also a clinical professor of pediatrics. He is the author of the popular book *ADHD Without Drugs: A Guide to the Natural Care of Children with ADHD.*

CHAPTER 12. OPIOIDS AND THE TREATMENT OF CHRONIC PAIN

Robert Bonakdar, MD, is director of pain management at the Scripps Center for Integrative Medicine in La Jolla, California, and assistant clinical professor at the University of California, San Diego School of Medicine. He is the coeditor of *Integrative Pain Management.*

CHAPTER 13. ANTIHYPERTENSIVE DRUGS

J. Adam Rindfleisch, MPhil, MD, is a family physician and associate professor at the University of Wisconsin Department of Family Medicine and Community Health. He has an integrative primary care practice and directs the University of Wisconsin's academic integrative medicine fellowship program.

CHAPTER 14. MEDICATIONS FOR DIABETES

Denise Millstine, MD, is an assistant professor of medicine and director of the integrative medicine program at the Mayo Clinic Hospital in Phoenix. She is also on the faculty of the University of Arizona Center for Integrative Medicine.

Chapter 15. Medications for Osteopenia and Other Preconditions

Elizabeth S. Smoots, MD (DrSmoots.com), practices family medicine in Seattle. She is the medical director for Practical Prevention, a program that helps health care businesses educate their clients about staying healthy, fit, and well. Dr. Smoots authored the popular book *Allergy Guide: Alternative and Conventional Solutions.*

Chapter 16. Overmedication of Children

Hilary McClafferty, MD, FAAP, is board certified in pediatrics, pediatric emergency medicine, and integrative medicine. She is associate professor in the Department of Medicine at the University of Arizona College of Medicine and director of the pediatric Integrative Medicine in Residency program at the University of Arizona Center for Integrative Medicine, where she also leads the fellowship in integrative medicine. She chairs the American Academy of Pediatrics' Section on Integrative Medicine and is the author of the upcoming book *Integrative Pediatrics: Art, Science, and Clinical Application.*

CHAPTER 17. OVERMEDICATION OF THE ELDERLY

Julia Jernberg, MD, completed a three-year geriatrics research fellowship at the University of Wisconsin. She has served on the geriatrics faculty of the University of Arizona and is currently medical director of the Iora Health geriatric medicine clinic in Tucson.

CHAPTER 18. OVER-RELIANCE ON MEDICATIONS: A PHARMACIST'S VIEW

Kim DeRhodes, BS, RPh, is a pharmacist practicing in Charlotte, North Carolina. She has over thirty-five years of experience in both hospital and retail pharmacy settings, with certification in medication therapy management. In addition, she is trained in the use of vitamins, herbs, and dietary supplements. She sees patients by appointment to review their medications and counsel them on the optimal use of supplements.

Hang M. (Emiley) Pham, PharmD, completed the Fellowship at the University of Arizona Center for Integrative Medicine. She currently works as a community pharmacist in El Cajon, California.

MIND
OVER
MEDS

Too Many Meds:
The Problem — and the Solution

We have a problem. More people are taking more medications than ever before and that is cause for concern. Use of prescription drugs has skyrocketed since the middle of the last century: Americans now take ten times as many as they did in the 1950s. About half of us are now taking at least one, an increase of over 20 percent just since 1994. Use of over-the-counter (OTC) medications has exploded just as dramatically. And more of us than ever are consuming dietary supplements, herbal remedies, and other products promoted for their health benefits, even though scientific evidence is often lacking for the safety and efficacy of many of them.

How many medications do you take? How about your parents? Your children? Your friends? Do you know what they're for? How they work? What their benefits and risks are? How they might interact—with one another and with other products you may be taking?

Whether there are alternatives to drugs to manage the health conditions you or your loved ones might have?

Too often, drugs fail to correct the problems they are meant to solve or simply reduce symptoms without addressing the root causes of disease. Too often, they are seen as quick and easy fixes for conditions that would be better addressed by changing dietary patterns, increasing physical activity, correcting sleep disturbances, and practicing techniques to neutralize the damaging effects of stress. At best, the benefits of many of the most widely used medications fall far short of the claims made by manufacturers, who also downplay their risks. At worst, many of those medications do more harm than good.

"All doctors do is give you pills" is a complaint I hear from many patients. More and more doctors tell me they are not comfortable with this. One recently told me she was "tired of being a pill pusher." Another, a psychiatrist, said he was dismayed that most psychiatric patients see a physician only four times a year—at a fifteen-minute appointment for adjustment of their medications.

In my role as director of the University of Arizona Center for Integrative Medicine I have taught hundreds of physicians, allied health professionals, medical residents, and students about the benefits and risks of drugs. One question I always ask is "How did we come to believe that medication is the only or the most effective way to treat disease?" *Medicine* and *medication* both derive from an ancient Indo-Iranian root meaning something like "thoughtful action to establish order"; the same root gives us the words *measure* and *meditate.* How curious that "thoughtful action" has become synonymous with the giving and taking of chemical substances.

Drugs are powerful. Some are miraculously effective— like opium and its derivatives for pain and antibiotics for bacterial infections that commonly killed throughout most of human history. The discovery of insulin saved many people with type 1 diabetes from an early death. Chemotherapy agents have cured forms of leukemia and lymphoma that had always been fatal. Antiviral drugs have turned HIV infection from a death sentence into a manageable chronic illness. No responsible physician today would reject medication as a method of treating disease and maintaining health.

But it is one method only. Many other interventions exist that do not involve drugs; sadly, they are not taught in conventional medical schools, and that is one reason that most doctors rely on medication. One example is dietary change. When I write a treatment plan for a patient, my first recommendations always concern diet: what not to eat, what to eat more of, how to change eating habits to improve health. As a primary treatment strategy, dietary change can be remarkably effective. Following an anti-inflammatory diet can so improve arthritis, allergies, and other conditions that medication can be reduced and in some cases eliminated. Much evidence links the Mediterranean diet with good health, longevity, and low risk of disease. The DASH diet is an effective intervention for lowering high blood pressure (DASH is an acronym for dietary approaches to stop hypertension). Eliminating cow's milk products from the diet often leads to marked improvement of recurrent ear infections in children and chronic sinusitis in adults. Eating whole soy foods regularly, beginning early in life, offers significant protection against hormonally driven cancers — breast cancer in women and prostate cancer in men. But because doctors are not trained in nutritional medicine, most of them are unable to give this sort of advice. Instead they rely on drugs.

Botanical remedies have been mainstays of folk medicine in many cultures throughout history. Many modern pharmaceutical drugs are derived from plants or are variations of molecules originally discovered in plants. Herbal medicines can be both safe and effective. For example, a freeze-dried preparation of the leaves of stinging nettle *(Urtica dioica)* relieves hay fever symptoms (itchy eyes, sneezing, runny nose) just as well as antihistamine drugs without any of their side effects. Extracts of the root of valerian *(Valeriana officinalis)* work well for many people to induce sleep. Extracts of the seeds of milk thistle *(Silybum marianum)* protect the liver from toxic injury (by alcohol, volatile solvents, and pharmaceutical drugs known to harm that organ). But because doctors are not trained in botanical medicine, most do not know how to use plant remedies. Instead they rely on drugs.

Mind-body medicine is a general term for therapies that take advantage of the connection between mind and body. These include hypnosis, guided imagery, visualization, biofeedback, meditation, and other techniques that are both cost and time effective. I frequently refer patients to practitioners of mind-body medicine and routinely see them bring about striking improvement and sometimes complete resolution of problems as diverse as atopic dermatitis (eczema), irritable bowel syndrome, and autoimmunity. But because none of this is in the conventional medical curriculum, most doctors do not know when and how to make such referrals. Instead they rely on drugs.

Breath work—learning how to change breathing habits and practicing specific breathing techniques—has remarkable effects on physiology. It cannot cause harm, requires no equipment, and costs nothing. It can correct some cardiac arrhythmias and gastrointestinal problems, for example, and is the most effective treatment I know for anxiety, as well as the simplest method of stress reduction. But because information on breath work is totally absent from conventional medical training, very few doctors can instruct patients about it. Instead they rely on drugs.

Evidence for the health benefits of exercise is

overwhelming. Increased physical activity can effectively prevent and treat depression, help normalize high blood pressure, and, along with dietary adjustment, put many cases of type 2 diabetes into complete remission. Doctors get some training here, but they are not trained in ways to motivate patients to exercise. Instead they rely on drugs.

Manual medicine, such as chiropractic and osteopathic manipulation and various forms of massage, is a safe and effective treatment, not just for musculoskeletal disorders but for other health conditions as well. Cranial therapy, an osteopathic technique, can end cycles of recurrent ear infections in children with none of the adverse effects of frequent courses of antibiotics. Visceral manipulation, also performed by some osteopathic physicians, can correct malfunctions of abdominal organs. But because most doctors are unfamiliar with manual medicine, they do not know when and how to refer patients to it. Instead they rely on drugs.

Traditional systems like Chinese medicine and Ayurveda comprise a variety of therapies, including dietary adjustment, herbal remedies, massage, and specialized techniques like acupuncture in Chinese medicine and detoxification regimens in Ayurveda. They can effectively manage some chronic health conditions, such as asthma, allergy, and inflammatory bowel disease. Acupuncture can dramatically improve acute sinusitis as well as reduce back pain and depression. But because doctors do not learn about these systems in their training, most do not know when to refer patients to them or how to find competent practitioners. Instead they rely on drugs.

The makers of those drugs, collectively known as Big Pharma, profoundly influence physicians. They fund research, which then drives practice. In the studies, drugs are measured against placebos to determine efficacy but almost never against lifestyle changes that may work as well or better. The information that doctors rely on when prescribing comes more often from industry sources than from objective ones. And despite attempts to curtail their influence, representatives of those companies are still very much present in medical offices, doing their best to persuade doctors to push their products. Pharmaceutical ads are the major revenue source for medical journals, compromising the objectivity of these journals in accepting or rejecting articles that report research findings with drugs and in deciding which to feature prominently.

Add to all this the strong desire of American patients to be medicated. Their belief in the power of drugs is as great as their physicians'. If the average doctor were told to manage a case without medication, he or she would likely not know what to do. If the average patient knew that no prescription would be forthcoming at the end of a medical visit, he or she would likely feel cheated and seek another practitioner to give one, especially for a product advertised on television. In recent years, direct-to-consumer advertising of prescription drugs has greatly increased consumer demand for them. New Zealand is the only country other than the United States that allows such promotion, which has been a boon for drug manufacturers and a disaster for medical practice.

Consider also that nondrug therapies require active participation of patients and may take more time to produce results. Lifestyle modification is particularly demanding. People will not change their eating habits or start exercising unless they are motivated to make the effort. Many patients would rather skip the effort and take a pill. The cost of the pill is often covered in whole or in part by insurance. There may be no reimbursement for dietary supplements, herbal remedies, or the nondrug therapies I have mentioned.

It's no wonder how we came to believe that medication is the only or the most effective way to treat disease.

So why is this cause for concern? Two reasons: the safety and the efficacy of the medications we rely on.

No difference exists between a drug and a poison except dose. (*Pharmacology* comes from the Greek word for poison.) All drugs become toxic as the dose is increased, and some poisons are in fact useful therapeutic agents at very low doses. Medicinal plants are usually much safer than their purified derivatives, because the active components are present in low concentrations, rarely more than 5 or 10 percent of the dry weight of the plant, and often less. Herbal remedies are dilute forms of natural drugs. Of course, they can be concentrated into liquid or solid extracts, but these products are still relatively low in potency compared to isolated purified compounds. And those compounds can be altered to make them even more potent—a favorite strategy of pharmaceutical chemists. The most widely used pharmaceutical drugs are extremely potent. Potent drugs may be necessary in cases of critical and severe illness, but we now use them for all disease conditions, even those that are not severe. Unfortunately, concentration of pharmaceutical power inevitably also concentrates toxicity; the two are inseparable.

Doctors have come to believe that the best medications are those that work quickly and powerfully. The consequence of reliance on such strong drugs is the very high incidence of adverse reactions to them that range from transient discomfort to permanent injury and death.

My own interest in learning how to treat common forms of illness without medication grew as I observed more and more cases of drug toxicity. One early experience I will never forget involved the death of a patient during my internship year at Mount Zion Hospital in San Francisco in 1969. On a month-long neurology rotation, I participated in morning rounds with two attending physicians and two medical residents. One day we saw a newly admitted patient who had suffered a massive stroke, a man in his late eighties. He was in a coma, unresponsive, with little chance of recovery. The immediate concern was that he was having frequent seizures, which soon became continuous. The senior attending physician was about to stop them with an intravenous dose of the tried-and-true anticonvulsant drug, phenytoin (Dilantin), but I spoke up to say that a lecturer at Harvard Medical School had told our class that intravenous diazepam (Valium), newly approved for treating continuous seizures, was superior. "Go ahead and try it," said the attending.

The rest of the team moved on. I asked a nurse to bring me a syringe of Valium and, following the directions on the product, slowly injected the appropriate dose into the patient's intravenous line. His seizures stopped within a minute. Pleased with myself, I left the room to rejoin the group. Minutes later, I received an emergency page. The drug had stopped not only the patient's seizures but also his breathing. He was dead from respiratory arrest.

No matter that he was moribund before I injected him with Valium or that he had a peaceful exit. I was devastated. Needless to say, I never again shot anyone up with Valium (nor with any other powerful pharmaceutical).

Hundreds of thousands of deaths occur each year in the United States as a result of adverse drug reactions. And we are not talking about medication errors here:

in these all-too-frequent cases, the right drug is given to the right patient in the right dose for the right indication. Adverse drug reactions are the fourth leading cause of death in our country and rank between the fourth and sixth most common cause of death in hospitalized patients.

The US Food and Drug Administration (FDA) requires manufacturers to disclose all possible adverse effects of drugs in labeling and advertising. Often these are so numerous that they take up most of the space in print ads. I have on my desk a three-page advertising spread from a national news magazine for brexpiprazole (Rexulti), headlined "It's time to feel better about facing the world." Rexulti is an antipsychotic drug, developed originally to treat major mental illness but now approved for treatment of depression in combination with antidepressant medications. (Studies increasingly show the most widely used antidepressants to be not that effective, but the combination is not much better. You can read about this questionable practice in chapter 9.) The ad exhorts people who have been on an antidepressant for at least eight weeks and are still feeling depressed to ask their doctors "if adding Rexulti is right for you." The fine print that fills most of the three pages describes the side effects and toxic calamities that can befall those who take the drug, including confusion, suicidal thoughts, uncontrolled body movements, metabolic problems, stroke, and death.

In television and radio ads for pharmaceuticals, announcers have to speak comically fast to list all the warnings and dire possibilities, an easy target for parody. But there is nothing funny about experiencing a severe adverse reaction to medication.

Keep in mind that all drugs have multiple effects on various organs and body functions. They are marketed, prescribed, and consumed for one desired effect, with the others relegated to fine print under the heading of "Possible Side Effects." But for some unlucky individuals, one of those side effects might turn out to be the main event. The most popular class of antidepressant medications—the selective serotonin reuptake inhibitors, or SSRIs—increase brain levels of the neurotransmitter serotonin. We tend to ignore the influences of these drugs on muscle and sexual function, unless those overwhelm any positive effects on mood. Antibiotics that we use to kill or inhibit the growth of disease-causing bacteria may alter liver and kidney function and interfere with digestion. A decision to take medication should take account of these risks, which are much greater than risks of lifestyle change and most nondrug therapies.

Consider, too, that individuals vary in how they respond to medication, a stubborn fact rarely emphasized in the training of physicians or in the marketing materials of drug manufacturers. For example, some people cannot tolerate statins, because they experience severe muscle pain or weakness from them. If significant numbers of people are affected by an adverse reaction, it is called a "side effect." If few are affected, it is an "idiosyncratic reaction" — that is, one peculiar to the individual. Variations in response to the same medication may reflect genetic differences or quirks of biochemistry. A new era of targeted drug therapy is on the horizon: genomic analysis may reveal who will respond positively to a drug and who will not. For now, most doctors' prescribing habits adopt a "one size fits all" mentality.

Do not assume that OTC medications are free of toxicity. They can cause serious adverse reactions on their own and can also interact with prescribed medications in ways that increase risk. Today, you can buy OTC forms of NSAIDs (nonsteroidal anti-inflammatory drugs), steroids, and the acid-blocking drugs indicated for GERD (gastroesophageal reflux disease). Their availability without a prescription encourages casual use without regard to the problems they can cause. As you will read in the pages that follow, it is also easy to get into trouble with popular OTC sleep aids and cold and flu remedies.

Many medical interventions (and many activities we choose to engage in) involve risk. The key is to determine the balance between risk and benefit. Immunization can cause harm, but to my mind and in the consensus opinion of medical science, the benefits of immunization greatly outweigh the risks. That is to say, the harm done by the diseases immunizations prevent is much greater than any harm done by immunizing. That may be small consolation to the parents of a child who suffers a severe adverse reaction to a vaccine, but it is nonetheless true.

I often ask doctors and medical students to compile a list of the medications they would take with them if they were going to live on a desert island. My list would include aspirin, penicillin, morphine, prednisone, and a few other drugs whose effectiveness in our collective experience is great enough to make for a favorable risk/benefit ratio. I would include none of the pharmaceutical products now so vigorously advertised on television, radio, and in print media. My general opinion of those is that manufacturers consistently exaggerate their benefits and consistently downplay the harm they can cause.

Drugs often appear to be most effective near the time of their introduction, becoming less so with the passage of time. Indeed, a much-quoted adage in medicine advises us to "use new medications as much as possible before they lose the power to heal." The reason has to do with the placebo response—healing from within initiated by belief in a drug or other treatment. Both doctors and patients tend to believe more in the power of new drugs, and that belief can add a halo of mind-generated efficacy to a drug's intrinsic action. I'm all for placebo responses; rather than trying to rule them out as most researchers want to do, we ought to be looking for ways to make them happen more often. After all, they represent the activity of the body's innate healing system. My preference is to elicit them not by deceiving patients with sugar pills but by presenting effective treatments with conviction, favoring gentler rather than harsher ones whenever possible. I would rather give less potent than more potent medications, always with the goal of increasing the likelihood of favorable responses and decreasing the likelihood of harm.

The SSRIs offer a case in point. When fluoxetine (Prozac) first came on the market in 1986, it was hailed as a breakthrough treatment for depression. In the years following, it and related medications were prescribed to millions of people. The effectiveness of SSRI antidepressants was documented in numerous randomized controlled trials (RCTs), the "gold standard" of scientific evidence for medical treatments. But by the turn of the twenty-first century, the power of SSRIs seemed to wane. Not only were there increasing reports of serious side effects and adverse reactions, it also became harder for researchers to distinguish response to SSRIs from that of placebo treatments. Enthusiasts for the drugs conceded that might be true in cases of mild depression, but they continued to believe in the value of SSRIs for moderate to severe depression. Further studies failed to demonstrate efficacy in moderate depression; the last holdouts still believe that they are useful for managing very severe depression. As the efficacy of SSRIs has steadily waned, the pharmaceutical companies have persuaded doctors to beef them up by combining them with other drugs, especially antipsychotics like Rexulti.

The fact is that all the regulations we have and all the testing we do, including RCTs, have not kept many worthless and dangerous drugs from coming on the market. Trials can be designed, data manipulated, and results interpreted to make new medications appear more effective than time and experience will prove them to be.

And even when medications work, they may not do what we want them to do. The bone-building drugs widely used to treat age-related loss of bone density (osteopenia) do increase bone mass, but how effective are they at preventing fractures, which is the benefit we want? As you will see in chapter 15, the answer is "not very." Statins are very effective at lowering LDL ("bad") cholesterol levels in blood, but does that translate to better health and reduced risk of heart attack? As you will find in chapter 2, the answer is "not necessarily."

Moreover, when used long term, many of the most widely prescribed medications can actually prolong or worsen the conditions they are meant to relieve. The reason has to do with homeostasis, a basic principle of physiology that designates a living organism's tendency to maintain equilibrium. (The word *homeostasis* derives from Greek roots, meaning "standing still.") If an external force disturbs the body's balance, the body reacts against it to regain balance. Reduce caloric intake and your body compensates by slowing metabolism—to the great frustration of dieters.

Most of our medications counteract or suppress aspects of physiology. You can quickly get a sense of this by considering the names of drug categories. We use antispasmodics, antihypertensives, antidepressants, anti-inflammatories, anti-this and anti-that. Strong counteractive medications are indeed useful for short-term management of health conditions resulting from severe imbalances of body function. When they are continued long term, however, especially without attention to the root causes of illness, they are likely to ensnare patients in the homeostatic trap. The body reacts against the pharmacological actions, making it difficult to lower dosage or discontinue medication because of rebound symptoms.

Put a patient with GERD on a drug that blocks acid production in the stomach and guess what? The body will try to make more acid, so that if the drug is discontinued, the symptoms of GERD come right back, often with a vengeance. In fact, if you put people without any gastric problems on one of these medications for a couple of months, then stop it abruptly, most will develop acid-related symptoms. And you can imagine the result of maintaining depressed patients on SSRIs.

The homeostatic reaction of the brain to the increased levels of serotonin they cause is to produce less of that neurotransmitter and fewer receptors for it, not only making it hard to get off the medication but also prolonging or intensifying the depression.

In the following chapters, you will learn about other examples of unintended consequences of reliance on medications that illustrate the body's natural tendency to resist disturbance. I'm afraid these are all too common today. They should motivate both doctors and patients to explore ways of managing chronic health conditions without relying solely on medications. Let me repeat that drug therapy can be lifesaving in cases of critical and acute illness and is an important component of treatment of chronic illness *in the context of comprehensive care that also includes lifestyle modification and nondrug therapies.* Long-term use of medications as stand-alone treatment, though, is simply not wise.

My reason for writing this book is simple. I believe that few people on popular medications understand how they work, whether they work well enough to justify the risks of using them, and what other effective methods of treatment are available to use along with them or in place of them. I began this project by drawing up a list of the categories of medications I find most concerning, the ones that are most overprescribed and misprescribed, overused and misused:

Antibiotics
Statins
Medications for GERD
Antihistamines
Medications for the Common Cold and the Flu
Sleep Aids
Steroids
NSAIDs
Psychiatric Medications
Medications for ADHD
Opioids
Antihypertensive Drugs
Medications for Diabetes
Medications for Osteopenia and Other
    Preconditions

Because I am not an expert in all these categories, I asked medical colleagues in appropriate specialties to help me gather and assess relevant information on them. Most of the contributors are graduate fellows or faculty members of the University of Arizona Center for Integrative Medicine in clinical practice. In addition, I asked a pediatrician to write about overmedication of children and an internist who works with older patients to provide data on overmedication of the elderly; I regard both as areas of concern. And, finally, I invited a pharmacist to write a chapter on her view of the overuse and misuse of medications.

Let me explain that last decision. Of all health professionals, pharmacists are the most knowledgeable about medications, OTC products as well as prescribed ones. They are trained to advise both doctors and patients about proper ways to use medications, including their possible interactions with one another. Sadly, pharmacists are underutilized for this purpose. (Ideally, they should also be able to give advice about herbal remedies, dietary supplements, and other natural products promoted for improving health and treating disease and to warn consumers about how they might interact with medications, but I find pharmacy education in this area to be deficient.) In chapter 18, Kim DeRhodes, RPh, explains how you can take advantage of a service pharmacists are trained to provide: a medication therapy management session to help you use medications wisely and avoid getting into trouble with them.

Each chapter includes one or two case presentations—stories of actual patients who experienced the problems these common classes of drugs too often cause. I will explain their actions, benefits, and risks. In addition, I will inform you about other ways of managing the conditions they are meant to treat and suggest what integrative treatment for those conditions might look like.

The consequences of overmedication go beyond adverse reactions, drug interactions, ineffectiveness, and unintended worsening of health problems. The cost of medicines, especially prescription products, is a huge burden, both on patients and families and on our failing health care system. The markup on pharmaceutical drugs is greater than on any other commodity in the marketplace. Big Pharma justifies this by citing the high cost of research, but what the companies spend on research is a small fraction of what they spend on advertising and promotion. If you are an American, you should also know that you pay much more for prescription drugs than people do in other countries— sometimes twice as much for the same product.

The expense of medications is often hidden in the modest copays of insurance plans, but you can be sure that the manufacturers get their money; in the end, we all pay. Per-person spending on drugs in our country is close to $1,000 annually, almost twice as much as per-person spending in other industrialized nations. US spending for prescription drugs is close to $300 billion per year—a significant contributor to the escalating cost of health care. In nearly every case, integrative treatment based on lifestyle modification and judicious use of natural products and nondrug therapies is less expensive than long-term medication treatment for common health conditions.

Much less attention is paid to the effects on the environment of all the medication being consumed. Many pharmaceutical products are neither digested nor changed in the body. They leave it and enter the environment, as do drugs that we flush down the toilet and those that wind up in landfill. They accumulate in water supplies, in soil, and in the foods we eat. We may be absorbing low levels of them constantly, but we have no data on how they might impact our health over a lifetime. We do know that a major cause of increasing resistance of bacteria to antibiotics—now a serious threat to public health—is the constant presence of those drugs in the environment, much of it from agricultural runoff. (Almost all animals we raise for food, including farmed fish, are put on antibiotics to promote growth.)

The information in these pages can help you become a wise consumer: to know whether pharmaceutical products are really needed, to be able to weigh their benefits against possible risks, to be wary of the persuasive efforts of Big Pharma. I want you to know, too, that many of the health conditions discussed in the following chapters can be managed without drugs or with integrative treatment plans that use fewer of them or less potent ones or lower dosages of them in combination with other methods.

When I was growing up in the late 1940s and 1950s, doctors wrote prescriptions in Latin in order to keep patients in the dark about medications. To fill a prescription, you had to hand it to a pharmacist who stood behind a high counter intended to prevent you from seeing what he did. Few patients asked questions about these practices. Of course, times have changed. The paternalistic and authoritarian style of doctors of the last century has gone out of fashion, and the Internet has made medical information available to anyone with access to a computer. In my opinion, however, people still do not ask enough questions about their medications, and that also contributes to the problem. Taking a drug just because a doctor says so is never a good idea. Always try to understand why you need it.

You might want to read this book from cover to cover, but please feel free to browse through it or use it as a reference work as needed. If you are on any of the medications I discuss, you will probably want to read about those first. If what you read makes you uneasy about staying on them, keep this advice in mind:

- Never stop taking a prescribed medication suddenly.
- It is always best to wean off medication gradually and under the supervision of a health professional.
- Never attempt to discontinue medication without first putting in place other measures to manage the condition being treated.

Physicians you consult may be unfamiliar with the nondrug treatments and integrative approaches suggested in these chapters. My colleagues and I are working to encourage doctors and allied health professionals to learn about them. If doctors you consult are not open to it, seek out practitioners trained in integrative medicine. (See the Resources section on page 329.)

A Note About Drug Names

Drugs are known by generic names and by trademarked brand names. When I write about a medication in this book, I first give the generic name in lowercase, followed by the capitalized brand name(s) in parentheses—for example, diazepam (Valium) and fluoxetine (Prozac). When branded medications go off patent, less expensive generic forms often become available.

1

Antibiotics

I've put antibiotics up front because their history provides a grim object lesson about the consequences of overuse and misuse of powerful medications.

Penicillin was isolated from a common mold in 1928, and people began treating infections with it in 1942. In short supply, it was first made available to the military and then, after the end of the Second World War, to the general public. A true miracle drug, it saved many lives. Over the next years, scientists discovered many more antibiotics, mostly natural products derived from molds and related organisms. In nature, fungi and bacteria compete for resources and territory; antibiotics are the chemical defenses that fungi have evolved against bacterial competitors. They either inhibit the growth of bacteria or kill them outright.

I have a vivid memory of my first experience with

penicillin at the age of five, when I was down with a bad case of strep throat. Our family doctor, a beloved general practitioner, made a house call to examine me and told my mother that he was prescribing the new wonder drug. It came into my home in the form of thin, yellow, mint-flavored tablets to be dissolved under the tongue every four hours. They had to be kept in the refrigerator and seemed magical to me as well as precious. Within forty-eight hours, all my throat discomfort and malaise were gone.

The discovery of antibiotics was a revolutionary advance in medicine. Early on, these new medications were spectacularly effective. Had we used them judiciously—reserving them for treatment of serious bacterial infections, they would still serve us well. Instead, we—and I include physicians, nurses, pharmacists, and patients here—have used them thoughtlessly and promiscuously. As a result, we have directed the evolution of bacteria in alarming ways, giving rise to resistant organisms that are also extremely virulent, like the notorious MRSA (methicillin-resistant *Staphylococcus aureus*). Antibiotic resistance is now so widespread that it is considered a major threat to public health. In many ways we are now in worse relationships with disease-causing bacteria than we were before we had antibiotics—a calamity entirely of our own making.

Let me present an illustrative case:

Shawna is a twenty-one-year-old woman who was suffering from what seemed to be a sinus infection. She visited her doctor, who prescribed two weeks of amoxicillin (a type of penicillin sold under the brand name Augmentin) for this presumed infection. After taking her third dose, Shawna broke out in copious itchy hives over her chest and back. She called her doctor, who told her she was likely allergic to that antibiotic and warned her not to take it again. He prescribed another, azithromycin (Zithromax), for the remainder of the two-week course. Over the last few days on that drug, Shawna developed diarrhea. She was told that this was not unexpected after a course of antibiotics and that it should resolve within a few days of finishing them.

The diarrhea, however, didn't go away. Instead, it worsened—so much so that Shawna had to go to the emergency room, where she was given IV fluids. She underwent numerous stool tests for various parasites and bacteria and was sent home on a course of another antibiotic, metronidazole (Flagyl), to treat any untoward microbes that may have been causing the problem. The next day, she noticed blood and mucus in her stool. In a panic, she contacted her doctor again, and was told by his nurse that this was likely nothing more than a result of rectal irritation from diarrhea.

Shawna didn't believe it; there was just too much blood. She returned to the emergency room, was found to be severely anemic, and was sent for a CT scan with contrast that showed she had pseudomembranous colitis—massive inflammation and bleeding in her colon. The doctors told her this was likely related to an infection with a dangerous organism, *Clostridium difficile* (known as *C. diff*), which can result from overuse of antibiotics. At that point, Shawna was given an even more powerful antibiotic, vancomycin (Vancocin), considered the most effective treatment for *C. diff.* Her symptoms resolved, only to return as soon as she stopped taking the drug. After numerous rounds of vancomycin, it was determined that she had recurrent *C. diff.* By that point, Shawna, who was 5 feet 7 inches tall, had lost nearly fifteen pounds, down to a mere ninety pounds.

Shawna's family then took her to an integrative medicine doctor, who started her on high doses of oral probiotics—beneficial organisms—including *Saccharomyces boulardii,* a yeast proven to be useful in cases of *C. diff* infection. The new doctor recommended removing all processed foods from her diet, particularly those that contained food additives that can be damaging to the digestive tract, like carrageenan and polysorbate 80, and recommended eliminating processed sugar and grains for two months to reduce digestive stress. She also referred Shawna to a gastroenterologist, who administered fecal microbial transplant (FMT), a cutting-edge treatment for digestive infections resistant to antibiotics. Shawna underwent four FMTs while taking immune-boosting herbs, including echinacea, reishi mushroom, and astragalus. The diarrhea finally stopped completely, and Shawna began to regain the weight she'd lost. Within six weeks, she felt strong again and was able to return to graduate school.

Though Shawna's case may sound extreme, it is, unfortunately, an increasingly common example of the downside of antibiotics. They often disrupt digestion and cause diarrhea in up to 30 percent of patients who take them. In most cases, symptoms are mild, clearing up soon after the person stops taking the medication. But in 15 to 20 percent of patients with antibiotic-associated diarrhea, the cause is *C. diff,* an "opportunistic" organism that proliferates when antibiotics kill off the good bacteria that normally keep it in check. Every year about 500,000 people in the United States acquire *C. diff* infections, almost all of them associated with antibiotic treatment; about 30,000 people die as a result.

Antibiotics are prescribed to prevent the progression of documented or presumed bacterial infections, including ear infections, strep throat, pneumonia, urinary tract infections, sexually transmitted diseases like syphilis and gonorrhea, Lyme disease and associated tick-borne co-infections, and acne. Sometimes, they are prescribed in the absence of an infection as a preventive measure, for instance, to prevent infection following surgery. They do not treat viruses.

Some of the most common classes of antibiotics include penicillins, cephalosporins, aminoglycosides, macrolides, sulfonamides, tetracyclines, and quinolones. The prescriber chooses a drug within a particular class to treat a suspected or documented bacterial infection, while taking into account additional factors such as a patient's age, history of allergies, and the presence of other health conditions.

Unfortunately, even when prescribed appropriately, antibiotics are not without serious drawbacks, as we shall see in the following sections.

The Problems with Antibiotics

Antibiotic Resistance

Antibiotic resistance develops when bacteria evolve the ability to neutralize a drug and continue to multiply in its presence. Whenever an antibiotic is used, it acts as a selective agent for bacteria that can resist it and survive to pass on their genes. This can happen very fast, because bacteria reproduce rapidly and can easily pass genetic mutations for antibiotic resistance to their next generations. The more extensively an antibiotic is used, the faster this occurs.

Resistance can develop without human action when

bacteria defend themselves from antibiotics produced by fungi and other bacteria. However, the current prevalence of resistant germs is due almost entirely to the overuse and abuse of antibiotics. Genes for resistance allow bacteria to survive and grow in the presence of one or more antibiotics. Because bacteria can collect multiple resistance traits over time, they can become immune to entire classes of antibiotics.

Doctors have been routinely prescribing antibiotics for minor bacterial infections, for the prevention of infections that may or may not occur, for traveler's diarrhea and other gastrointestinal ailments, for the long-term treatment—often for years—of acne, rosacea, and other conditions that may or may not have a component of bacterial infection, and, worst of all, for viral illnesses, in which antibiotic therapy is pointless. Patients with viral upper respiratory infections commonly demand antibiotics when they do not get better quickly, and too often doctors comply. The body becomes a factory for generating resistant organisms that go out into the world to cause trouble for all of us—a consequence that is particularly regrettable when the use of the drug is not justified. In 2009, Americans spent almost $11 billion on antibiotic therapy. Resistant infections now account for $20 billion in annual health care costs.

Antibiotic exposure that promotes resistance can come from other sources as well. These medications are applied directly to crops as pesticides and also administered daily to livestock as growth promoters. Indeed, livestock consumed a whopping 32 million pounds of antibiotics in 2012 — more than four times the amount used in humans. Treated animals are raised in crowded, unhealthy conditions, then slaughtered and processed en masse. Resistant bacteria escape farms by way of the workers, their families, and the manure that is used to fertilize crops and can contaminate produce as well as waterways through runoff. Of the *Salmonella* bacteria that commonly show up in the US meat supply, 5 percent are now resistant to five or more classes of antibiotics, and 3 percent can withstand ceftriaxone (Rocephin), the current first-line therapy for salmonellosis in children. Residues of antibiotics are found in conventionally raised meat, poultry, milk and milk products, and farmed fish. (Recently, in response to growing concern, some fast-food restaurant chains have pledged to buy only antibiotic-free beef.)

Toxicity

Toxic effects of antibiotics vary with the class and range from mild to life threatening. Penicillins and cephalosporins are associated with rash and diarrhea, while aminoglycoside use can result in loss of hearing and kidney damage. Macrolides, such as erythromycin, commonly cause nausea and abdominal pain; tetracyclines can discolor the teeth of young children;

and sulfa drugs cause sun sensitivity. The quinolones can cause inflammation of the eyes, sun sensitivity, insomnia, fatigue, and in rare instances tendon rupture. They are also more likely to be associated with severe diarrheal disease due to *C. diff.*

Allergic Reactions

Antibiotic allergies are one of the most common drug allergies among both adults and children. These reactions affect about one in fifteen people, with penicillins and cephalosporins being the most common triggers. Antibiotic allergy may occur in the form of immediate or delayed reactions. The former are marked by lip or facial swelling, hives, itchy throat, vomiting, and, occasionally and most seriously, anaphylaxis (allergic shock). The symptoms of delayed antibiotic allergy are quite variable, including skin redness, rash or swelling, organ dysfunction (hepatitis, nephritis), and blood abnormalities. The most severe forms of delayed reactions can be life threatening.

Sometimes, an antibiotic allergy occurs in response to an unexpected exposure. One published study described the case of a Canadian girl who experienced facial flushing, hives, and abnormal breathing shortly after eating a slice of blueberry pie. She was taken to an emergency room, treated with epinephrine and other drugs, and recovered. A team of doctors then investigated what might have caused the girl's reaction.

Although the patient was allergic to milk, an analysis showed that the pie did not contain milk. Tests for all the other ingredients in the pie also came back negative, but further analysis showed the presence of an antibiotic. The doctors tested the girl for an allergy to streptomycin, an antibiotic used as a pesticide on fruit. And, indeed, she reacted to it in much the same way as she had responded to the blueberry pie. Allergic reactions to antibiotic residues in food are underdiagnosed, because their presence is not noted on product labels. If doctors suspect them, they must send a food sample to a specialized laboratory for analysis.

Damage to the Microbiome

There are ten times more bacterial cells than there are "human" cells in our bodies, most of them concentrated in the intestines. Those bacteria help us digest food and synthesize vitamins. They also help fortify our defenses against germs that can cause infections and influence our health, both physical and mental, in many other ways. Antibiotics upset the body's balance of gut microbes, conceivably preventing the immune system from accurately distinguishing between harmless compounds and real attacks. A poorly balanced gut flora can make the mucosal lining more permeable, allowing large molecules that normally stay within the gut to leak into the systemic circulation, which in turn induces immune responses that might lead to allergy and autoimmunity.

One research team fed mice a species of yeast commonly found on human skin, after treating some of them with a course of an antibiotic. Usually, this yeast is not able to live in mice, but because the antibiotic suppressed natural gut bacteria, the yeast became established in the treated mice (similar to the way a vaginal yeast infection can develop after women start a course of antibiotics). Over the course of the following two weeks, the researchers exposed all the mice to inhaled fungal spores that typically trigger an allergic response. Those that had received the antibiotic reacted much more strongly to the spores, presumably as a result of their altered gut flora. This finding suggests that changes in the composition of the gut microbiome following antibiotic treatment can make us more susceptible to respiratory and other allergies. A lack of healthy gut bacteria has also been associated with inflammatory bowel disease and even cancer.

A 2011 article in the journal *Nature* states that changes in the microbiome may facilitate the transmission of dangerous germs, noting that one of the important roles of normal gut flora is to resist colonization by pathogenic organisms. Not only do antibiotics cause permanent changes in the gut flora, but infants born to women given antibiotics during pregnancy, as well as the 30 percent of American children delivered via cesarean section, may be starting life with an abnormal microbiome. This is of concern because lack of diversity in friendly gut bacteria has been shown to contribute to a large number of diseases and complications. Even a single course of antibiotics can permanently alter the gut flora. One study found that after a single treatment with intravenous antibiotics, fecal bacteria tests demonstrated a significant change in the variety of bacterial strains, as well as the presence and growth of *C. difficile*.

Changes in the microbiome due to antibiotics have even been linked with obesity. Gut bacteria present in obese subjects differ significantly in species type from those found in lean subjects. Low-calorie diets, where either fat or carbohydrates are restricted, change the gut flora and increase the abundance of the bacterial strains found more commonly in lean subjects. It appears that certain types of gut flora are associated with obesity because they extract energy from food more efficiently.

Mitochondrial Damage

Called the "powerhouses" of the cell, mitochondria produce energy essential for cells of both plants and animals to function. Mitochondria are thought to be ancient bacteria that evolved to become a critical part of the cellular apparatus. It's not surprising, then, that several studies have found that commonly prescribed antibiotics such as doxycycline, ampicillin, ciprofloxacin, levofloxacin, and an entire class called beta-lactams can have detrimental impact on mitochondrial function. Some impair mechanisms that protect mitochondria from oxidative damage. Others alter mitochondrial DNA. Although the consequences in humans are unclear, scientists have observed disturbed growth of common plants transplanted from untreated soil to soil with varying concentrations of doxycycline. They noted "delays in growth, some quite severe" after just a few days, even in soils in which the concentration of the antibiotic was about that found in some agricultural soils today. The delays appeared to be due to mitochondrial dysfunction.

INTEGRATIVE MEDICINE APPROACHES TO PREVENTING AND TREATING INFECTION

Some of the most effective approaches to avoiding transmissible infectious illness are deceptively easy, including washing your hands with soap and staying home when you're sick (or keeping an ill child home). Isolating yourself until you feel well not only reduces your chance of exposing others when you're most contagious but also allows you to rest and recover faster.

You are most often exposed to microbes when you

touch your eyes, nose, or mouth after touching a contaminated surface. Though you may not think of yourself as much of a face-toucher, researchers at the University of California at Berkeley found that people touch their eyes, nose, and mouth an average of 15.7 times per hour. Scrubbing your hands with plain old soap and warm water for twenty seconds works as well as applying hand sanitizer to prevent infection — and more so if your hands are greasy or caked in dirt. Indeed, in 2016 the US Food and Drug Administration banned the use of certain antibacterial chemicals in the use of hand soaps amid concerns about both their safety and efficacy.

For disinfecting surfaces, bleach may not offer as much protection as we had thought. A study of children in the Netherlands, Finland, and Spain who were regularly exposed to bleach-cleaned environments had higher rates of respiratory tract infections, including influenza, bronchitis, and tonsillitis, than those who lived in homes where disinfectant cleaners were not used. In fact, many experts consider over-sanitizing a big mistake. Applying germicidal chemicals in the home, the workplace, and public spaces selects for more virulent organisms and probably weakens immunity. That possibility follows from the "hygiene hypothesis," which argues that the immune system gains strength and experience from regular exposure to germs early in life. Children who grow up in too-clean environments have higher rates of allergy and asthma and may be more susceptible to infection than children who have pets, are raised on farms, or play in the dirt.

Research is telling us that the long-held belief that all microbes are dangerous is far from correct. The bacteria, viruses, fungi, and even parasites that live on us and in us keep one another in balance. It can indeed be dangerous or even deadly for any one microbial population to multiply unchecked. But while we previously thought that the answer was to sanitize—our bodies with antibiotics and hand sanitizers and our environments with bleach and other disinfectants—it turns out that constant exposure to an array of biodiverse microorganisms is an effective defense against infection that may also reduce risks of allergy, autoimmune disease, and other health problems. From all we're learning, a body that's rich in microbial diversity is more resilient.

Probiotics are beneficial microorganisms that, when administered in adequate amounts, confer health benefits. A variety of bacteria have been studied to explore their probiotic effect, including *Lactobacillus rhamnosus* GG, other species of *Lactobacillus* and *Bifidobacterium,* and the yeast *Saccharomyces boulardii.* A review of thirty-one randomized studies found that when probiotic supplements are given along with antibiotics, they reduce the risk of developing digestive symptoms—including *C. difficile* diarrheal illness—by 64 percent. Regular consumption of probiotic-rich foods can also be helpful, possibly more so than taking supplements. These include sauerkraut, kimchi, and pickles—the live-culture versions that have to be refrigerated—as well as yogurt (containing live active cultures), kefir, and miso. Organic fruits and vegetables that are not power-washed provide traces of beneficial soil flora. And several studies show that spending sustained time in the forest boosts immune function.

Foods that have clear immune-boosting properties include those that contain bitter compounds, such as dark leafy greens, the peel on certain vegetables and fruits, coffee, and even dark chocolate. These protective phytonutrients enhance immunity not only in the digestive tract, which can help prevent infection there, but also in the ear, nose, and throat, thereby increasing defenses against colds, sore throat, and flu. Raw, unprocessed honey also can boost immunity in older children and adults and prevent wound infection; these benefits spring from plant polyphenols and other compounds in flower nectars as well as from the presence of a particular probiotic organism, *Lactobacillus kunkeei*, which is endemic among honeybees.

Some botanicals can also boost immunity and help prevent infection, such as astragalus *(Astragalus membranaceus)*, echinacea *(Echinacea* spp.), and elderberry

(Sambucus nigra). So can medicinal mushrooms like turkey tail *(Trametes versicolor),* reishi *(Ganoderma lucidum),* maitake *(Grifola frondosa),* and shiitake *(Lentinula edodes).* Thyme and sage, as extracts or infusions in honey, also have antimicrobial properties. Studies done on essential oils of eucalyptus, tea tree, lemongrass, and others have shown these to be selectively effective against various types of bacteria, including famously resistant ones like MRSA.

BOTTOM LINE

Antibiotics can be critically important for people with overwhelming bacterial infections. They have saved countless lives. No matter the benefits, however, we must take into account their detrimental impacts on short- and long-term health.

Experts warn that we are coming to the end of the antibiotic era, as bacteria have now developed resistance to our latest and strongest drugs. The appearance of new "superbugs" may force us to explore other ways of preventing and fighting infection, such as reviving treatment protocols from the days before we had antibiotics: aggressive cleaning and disinfecting of wounds, for instance, and relying again on older medications, such as boric acid, phenol, and preparations of silver.

Alternative approaches are important for decreasing

not just human use of antibiotics but also their use in food production, which would dramatically reduce exposure and might slow the development of resistance and the appearance of potentially deadly strains.

For now, please heed this advice:

• Reserve antibiotics for treatment of severe bacterial infections.

• Never take an antibiotic for an upper respiratory infection (URI) that is likely to be viral in origin, even if symptoms are severe and persistent (in which case you should speak with your doctor), unless a throat culture or other test indicates the presence of pathogenic bacteria. Do not pressure your doctor to prescribe an antibiotic for an ordinary URI.

• Do not go on long-term antibiotic therapy for management of chronic skin, gastrointestinal, or respiratory ailments without carefully assessing the benefit/risk ratio.

• If you eat meat, poultry, dairy products, or farmed fish, choose organic versions or ones certified to be free of antibiotics.

• Build and protect immunity by getting adequate physical activity, sleep, and rest; by learning and practicing methods to neutralize the harmful effects of stress; by minimizing exposure to toxins (second-hand smoke, pesticides and other poisons, contaminated water, and so on); and by eating a balanced diet rich in protective compounds from vegetables, fruits, herbs, and spices.

• Make use of natural products that increase resistance to infection, such as astragalus and the Asian mushrooms mentioned above.

• Also learn to use natural products that are safe and effective treatments for minor infections, like tea tree oil *(Melaleuca alternifolia)* for skin and periodontal problems and Oregon grape root *(Mahonia aquifolium)* for the gastrointestinal tract.

2

Statins

We should put statins in the water supply." I can't count the times I have heard doctors say this, and I can hardly imagine a more wrong-headed idea. It represents a great lack of understanding of the effects of these powerful drugs and their risks versus benefits.

Here are the stories of two patients on statin therapy.

Janice is a sixty-two-year-old financial analyst with no health problems apart from a history of elevated cholesterol first noticed five years ago. She is careful about her diet — eats lots of vegetables and fruit, very little snack food, and chicken or beef only once a week. Janice exercises every other day at her health club and goes to yoga class once a week. Three years ago, her internist became concerned when her total cholesterol rose to 225 mg/dL and prescribed the cholesterol medicine simvastatin (Zocor). Follow-up labs six weeks later were normal, with a drop in total cholesterol to 165 mg/dL.

At a return visit six months later, Janice felt a bit less energetic than usual and said she had cut back on the intensity of her exercise program. One year later, at her annual checkup, she described feeling "older," with aching legs and "arthritis pains" in her elbows and wrists. Shortly thereafter, her husband took her on a surprise anniversary trip to Italy; in the excitement of preparing for the trip, she forgot to pack her simvastatin. While in Italy, her pain disappeared, as did the achiness in her legs.

Upon her return home, Janice decided not to restart the simvastatin. She has remained pain free. Although her total cholesterol is high, so is her "good" HDL cholesterol, and her overall risk of cardiovascular disease is low.

Jim, age fifty-six, is in the emergency room because of chest pain and is informed that he is having a heart attack, his second. At the time of his first, two years ago, his cholesterol was elevated and a statin was prescribed. Although Jim was initially reluctant to take cholesterol-lowering medication, his doctor convinced him that he wouldn't have to worry about his diet if he took a statin. Since the first heart attack, he has continued the medication but has not appreciably changed his eating habits. He wonders how he could be back in the hospital with another heart attack despite having faithfully taken a statin every day.

No class of drugs has been as venerated as the statins. Doctors have sung their praises since they first became available in the late 1980s. More recently, however, their detractors have been increasingly vocal.

In 1910, it was discovered that plaques in diseased arteries contain up to twenty times the amount of cholesterol found in normal blood vessels. These sticky lesions are also called *atheromas,* the Greek word for porridge. In the 1950s, a large study of the population of Framingham, Massachusetts, confirmed a link between high levels of cholesterol in the bloodstream and death from heart disease. Cholesterol circulates in blood in several forms, all bound to complexes of protein molecules, or lipoproteins. One form—high-density lipoprotein (HDL)—is known as "good" cholesterol, because it takes cholesterol from arteries and delivers it to the liver for excretion in bile. Low-density lipoprotein (LDL) is the "bad" form that deposits in arterial walls. There are also subtypes of HDL and LDL cholesterol associated with greater or lesser cardiac risk. Small, dense LDL particles, for example, are more dangerous than large, fluffy ones. A routine blood test today measures total cholesterol, LDL, HDL, and the LDL/HDL ratio (a higher number indicates higher risk of heart disease).

Nearly every cell in the human body can make

cholesterol, an essential component of cell membranes and the precursor for the biosynthesis of vitamin D, steroid hormones, and bile acids. Making cholesterol involves an intricate set of chemical pathways requiring more than thirty enzymes. Work began in the 1950s to identify compounds that could interfere with these pathways. In 1978, a potent blocker of one of the key enzymes in cholesterol production, HMG-CoA reductase, was discovered in the byproducts of a fermented fungus. This was the first statin.

In 1987, the US Food and Drug Administration (FDA) approved lovastatin (Mevacor) for human use. Since then, nearly a dozen different statins have been marketed—each with a slightly different chemical twist that alters its effect. In addition to lovastatin, the list of FDA-approved statins includes simvastatin (Zocor), fluvastatin (Lescol), pravastatin (Pravachol), atorvastatin (Lipitor), rosuvastatin (Crestor), and pitavastatin (Livalo). All but rosuvastatin and pitavastatin are currently available as less-expensive generics.

Some, like simvastatin, remain in the bloodstream for only a few hours before being broken down in the liver. Others, like atorvastatin and rosuvastatin, remain in the bloodstream much longer. The body makes most of its cholesterol at night while we sleep. For that reason, the shorter-acting statins, like simvastatin, need to be taken in the evening to maximize their effect.

Timing is not so important with the longer-acting drugs.

Most statins are degraded in the liver, where each type is slotted to a specific elimination path. Things can get complicated when several medications are taken together, as many drugs compete for the same chemical exit. This can cause the removal process to stall, leading to excessive buildup of a statin in the bloodstream and a higher risk of adverse effects.

A recent survey shows that a whopping 26 percent of adults in the United States are now taking a statin, at an annual cost to the health care system of more than $20 billion. And that number is expected to ratchet up even more based on the latest set of cholesterol guidelines from the American College of Cardiology/American Heart Association. According to these, as many as half of all adult Americans are candidates for statin therapy.

So are many children, according to pediatric guidelines that now call for drug treatment in children as young as ten years old with risk factors and only moderately elevated cholesterol. Inherited factors can cause total cholesterol levels to rise to over 500 mg/dL in children; those relatively rare conditions certainly warrant aggressive therapy because of their poor outlook. But, for the rest, it seems absurd to try to medicate away problems rooted in poor diet and inactivity. Not only is there a lack of evidence to support the extension of statin treatment to children, it sends the wrong message. Pills are not the answer for lifestyle-related problems—a truth we must help our children understand.

The ability of statins to lower LDL cholesterol is irrefutable. Depending on the product and dose, statins can reduce the LDL level by 30 to 50 percent. Whether or not drug-induced lowering of this form of cholesterol leads to better health, however, is a subject for debate.

(Although the benefits of statins are related to their cholesterol-lowering properties, new evidence suggests that other modes of action may be at work as well. One of particular interest is their role as anti-inflammatory agents. We now understand that inflammation plays a pivotal role in the development of vascular disease. Inflammatory cells are summoned to the site of cholesterol-laden plaques, where they weaken the delicate cap that encases the plaque, increasing the risk of a heart attack. Statins reduce the inflammatory response and thus help protect the "fault lines" within plaques from catastrophic fracturing.)

WHO BENEFITS MOST?

Two groups of people can potentially benefit from statin therapy: those who are at high risk of a heart attack based on their medical history, and patients with known vascular disease—including a history of heart attack, stroke, or poor circulation in the legs.

For those who have never had heart disease, the major risk factors for a heart attack include extremely high cholesterol levels (LDL cholesterol greater than 190 mg/dL), diabetes, a strong family history of heart disease, or a combination of other medical problems including high blood pressure and smoking.

The newest cholesterol guidelines include a "risk calculator" that estimates everyone's ten-year risk of heart disease or stroke to assess eligibility for statin treatment. Although this calculation has merit as an indicator of cardiovascular health status, an unfavorable risk assessment is better interpreted as a wake-up call to tackle lifestyle issues—in particular, diet, physical activity, and stress—than as a threshold for prescribing medication. Apart from age and family history, every one of the risk factors is exquisitely sensitive to lifestyle changes, such as adopting an anti-inflammatory diet and increasing exercise. Statins should be considered a last resort, and only for those whose risk factors can't be lowered to an acceptable level through lifestyle modification.

Even for people who need them, relying on statins too heavily can be problematic.

Let's put the benefits into perspective. In the best studies, statins reduce the chance of a heart attack in those at risk by no more than one-third. That's certainly a benefit that we should take advantage of, but it leaves two-thirds of the risk still on the table. That means that, given one hundred people destined to have a heart attack, statins would be expected to protect no more than thirty-three of them, while sixty-seven others would go on to have a heart attack despite taking the drugs.

The limitation of statin use in the absence of lifestyle changes is well illustrated by the second case above. Jim took his statin every day but did not change his diet, level of physical activity, or stress and went on to suffer a second heart attack—a scenario that happens all too often.

The Problems with Statins

Although statins have a place in the treatment of high-risk patients, they can have significant, and often overlooked, consequences. The spectrum of potential adverse effects ranges from muscle aches and weakness to cognitive impairment, diabetes, and liver dysfunction. Manufacturers of these drugs and their enthusiastic proponents tend to minimize, and sometimes ignore, these problems.

Muscle Pain

Pharmaceutical companies report a very low rate of muscle-related side effects from statins, ranging from 1 to 5 percent of patients. But many patients and physicians give a very different picture. Statin-induced muscle pain is one of the most common drug side effects in all of clinical medicine. In one recent study, 25 percent of individuals on statin therapy experienced it.

Because muscle pain is so common, it can be difficult to sort out whether a new ache is caused by a statin or by something else. But all too often, patients who suspect a statin-related problem don't even get the benefit of the doubt. A study of how physicians react to these complaints was revealing: among patients who reported muscle symptoms, 47 percent of the time physicians immediately dismissed the possibility that the drug was to blame.

These symptoms typically develop within the first month of use. However, their onset can range from a few days to several months, a time lag that can obscure the connection between symptoms and statin use. For some, the muscle problem develops quickly and with a vengeance, leaving little room for doubt that the medication is to blame. For others, like Janice described at the beginning of the chapter, the symptoms are insidious, slow to develop, and frequently mistaken for age-related changes.

In rare cases, statins can cause life-threatening muscle damage—rhabdomyolysis—leading to liver and kidney failure. This is more likely to happen with very high doses and interactions with other drugs.

Cognitive Impairment

Statins can also affect brain function. The list of cognitive problems linked to their use includes cloudy thinking, memory deficits, and depression. Of course, these symptoms are common in an aging population, and older people are more likely to be on statin therapy. The association of cognitive problems with statin use may be coincidental. Regardless, in many patients the problems resolve quickly once the drug is discontinued.

Unfortunately, there is no specific test to identify statins as the cause of cognitive decline. The only way to sort it out is to stop the drug for a few weeks and check for improvement. If cloudy thinking or memory impairment dissipates substantially, the statin is likely to blame. No major improvement suggests another cause.

Increased Risk of Diabetes

We already face a public health crisis: 50 percent of Americans are now either diabetic or pre-diabetic. It is especially concerning that statins could be contributing to this epidemic.

To keep this in perspective, know that only one new case of statin-induced diabetes will occur among 250 patients after four years of treatment. But given the magnitude of current statin use—in more than 40 million Americans—even a small increase in risk is significant.

For people at high risk of a heart attack, especially those who already have vascular disease, the benefit of taking a statin outweighs the risk of diabetes. A bigger problem arises, however, when statins are prescribed to those at low risk, in whom the potential for benefit is exceedingly small and the chance of inducing diabetes is not trivial. For people at low risk of heart disease, the overzealous use of statins may cause more illness than it prevents.

Liver Irritation

The liver is responsible for the breakdown and elimination of statins. This process occasionally overworks the organ, causing irritation indicated by elevation of liver enzymes in the blood. Typically, this side effect is inconsequential, but serious liver problems from statins have been reported. Before they are prescribed, blood tests are run to make sure the liver is healthy, and these may be repeated at intervals once the drug is started. If liver function tests suggest a problem, the dose may be lowered or even discontinued. If you are on a statin, you can reduce the risk of liver dysfunction by limiting your intake of alcohol and working with your health provider to trim your use of other medications that tax the liver.

Tips to Help Deal with Statin Side Effects

The development of a suspected statin side effect is a good opportunity to revisit the need for a statin in the first place. Those at lower risk might look to their health providers for alternative prevention options, including intensification of lifestyle efforts.

If a statin needs to be continued, a number of strategies can be useful to minimize side effects. It's important to know that different statins behave differently in the body, and each individual responds differently. Sometimes, switching to another statin or to a lower dose is all that's needed. (Some statins can be taken every other day or even twice a week to reduce side effects.)

It turns out that grapefruit contains a chemical that blocks a key pathway used by the liver to rid itself of certain statins, especially lovastatin, atorvastatin, and simvastatin. People on these medications should limit their intake of grapefruit and grapefruit juice to avoid high drug levels and associated side effects.

Milk thistle *(Silybum marianum)* is a safe botanical remedy that protects the liver from toxic injury. It can be taken along with a statin by those who experience liver irritation or have a history of liver disease.

A supplement that might help manage statin side

effects is coenzyme Q10, abbreviated CoQ10. The body makes this compound and uses it to produce ATP, the most important source of energy for cells, including muscle cells. Statins lower the level of CoQ10 in the blood, which may explain the muscle pain and other side effects of these drugs.

Several small studies have examined the use of CoQ10 supplements in statin-treated patients. Although some CoQ10 studies have shown an improvement in statin side effects, most have not. Nevertheless, many anecdotal reports describe benefit. Since the safety profile of CoQ10 is excellent, I believe that supplementation may well be worth a try when statin side effects are suspected. The usual dose is 60 to 100 milligrams twice a day of a softgel form taken with a fat-containing meal to ensure absorption.

Certain metabolic issues can also trigger statin-related problems. Vitamin D deficiency impacts cellular function on multiple levels and can thus lower the threshold for statin side effects. Replenishment of low vitamin D levels through supplementation can completely eliminate adverse reactions for some. I recommend 2000 IU a day for most people. If you have not had your blood level of vitamin D measured, do so: you may need to take higher doses initially if it is very low.

An underactive thyroid also increases the likelihood of statin-related problems. Diagnosis of this is easy to miss, however, because symptoms are vague and common with age: fatigue, intolerance to cold, and dry skin, for example. Blood tests for thyroid function should be checked when statin side effects are suspected.

INTEGRATIVE MEDICINE APPROACHES TO MANAGING HIGH CHOLESTEROL

An integrative approach to heart health goes beyond medication alone to take a wide-angle view of prevention. It begins with an anti-inflammatory diet, with abundant servings of vegetables, fruit, legumes, nuts, whole grains, less red meat and more fish, and high-quality extra-virgin olive oil.

Regular physical activity is essential for maintaining heart health. Even modest activity helps — as little as thirty minutes of walking every day has a sizeable impact. For those who are overweight, it's comforting to know that even when an exercise program does not lead to weight loss, it still appreciably lowers the odds of a heart attack.

Optimal heart health depends upon balance of the mind-body connection. Stress, anger, anxiety, and depression accelerate coronary disease, while optimism and gratitude are balms for the heart. Fortunately, positive moods and emotions can be cultivated.

Breath work offers a unique access to the involuntary nervous system and is a powerful method of relaxation. One very effective technique is the 4-7-8 breathing exercise: inhale for 4 counts, hold for 7 counts, then exhale for 8 counts. Repeat this sequence several times throughout the day. (A video showing the practice can be found at DrWeil.com.) Meditation is also remarkably beneficial, as documented in a study showing that regular practice reduces the likelihood of a cardiac emergency by 48 percent.

For those who cannot get their cholesterol level down enough through lifestyle change and also cannot tolerate prescription statins, a supplement called red yeast rice can be effective. Red yeast rice is a fermentation product of the yeast *Monascus purpureus* that has been used for centuries in China as an ingredient in food, mainly to add red color but also for its perceived health benefits. It contains several cholesterol-lowering compounds, all of which share the chemical structure of statins. (Interestingly, one of them, monacolin K, is the same compound as the first FDA-approved prescription statin, lovastatin.)

Although red yeast rice can cause the same side effects as prescription statins, it is much less likely to do so, probably because the body tolerates the natural mixture of similar molecules better than a single one. (The reason for this is not clear, but it is a pattern I observe with other complex natural products compared to purified pharmaceuticals.) In a randomized trial, 85 percent of patients who could not tolerate prescription statins were able to take red yeast rice without side effects. The trade-off with red yeast rice, however, is lower potency. The usual doses (1200 to 2400 mg/day) reduce LDL cholesterol by 20 to 25 percent, compared to 30 to 55 percent for prescription statins. It is available over the counter, and the recommended starting dose is 600 milligrams twice a day with food.

Other products that can help lower cholesterol include fiber, especially psyllium husk, as well as plant stanols and sterols that slightly reduce the amount of cholesterol absorbed from food. These are found in fruits, vegetables, legumes, nuts, and seeds, as well as fortified foods (some brands of orange juice, cereal, and granola bars). They are also available as dietary supplements.

BOTTOM LINE

Medication alone affords only limited protection against heart disease. Statins are very effective at decreasing LDL cholesterol, but that is only one of many risk factors. We would also like to able to raise HDL cholesterol and change the size of LDL particles, but we have no drugs to do that. Furthermore, half of those who have a first heart attack have *normal* blood cholesterol levels. Stress, anger, a sedentary lifestyle, and a diet that favors inflammation also predispose to blockages of coronary arteries. Too many doctors think they can deal with patients at risk for heart disease simply by prescribing a statin, ignoring its complex causes.

Based on the foundation of nutrition and lifestyle, an integrative approach to heart health recognizes the value of statins. But because these drugs have the limited effect of lowering LDL cholesterol and are not risk-free, judicious use is warranted. Current emphasis on statin therapy should be balanced by equal emphasis on lifestyle changes.

To put it bluntly: statins are no panacea and they do not belong in our drinking water.

3

Medications for GERD

Of all the medications covered in these pages, I am most concerned about the widespread, enthusiastic, reckless dispensing and consuming of drugs used to treat gastroesophageal reflux disease (GERD).

When I was growing up, GERD did not exist. People had heartburn, which they relieved with simple, safe antacids like Tums—chewable, mint-flavored tablets of calcium carbonate (that is, chalk). Most sufferers understood that heartburn is the stomach's way of letting you know you mistreated it: by eating too much, eating the wrong foods or combinations of foods, or not paying attention to the disruptive effects of stress and negative emotions on digestion. The goal is to correct those habits, not to suppress the symptom so that you can keep them up.

Now, heartburn has been medicalized, with total focus on overproduction of stomach acid as the primary problem and treatment with acid-blocking drugs as the primary intervention. Acid (and the enzymes it activates) in gastric secretions can irritate the lining of the stomach and lower esophagus, causing the pain and other symptoms of GERD, but except in very rare circumstances, overproduction of acid is not to blame. Moreover, adequate acid in the stomach facilitates digestion of protein and absorption of key vitamins (B_{12}) and minerals (calcium, iron, magnesium). It is also an important defense against infection, because strong acid kills potentially harmful bacteria and viruses. Trying to manage GERD solely by blocking acid production in the stomach without attending to the many other factors involved is not a wise strategy, especially in the long term.

Acid-blocking drugs are now some of the most widely sold medications worldwide. In the United States they have been among the top ten best-selling classes of medications since 2000. The first to come on the market were the H2 blockers—drugs that block histamine receptors, which are part of the acid production pathway in specialized cells in the stomach. Cimetidine (Tagamet) was approved in 1979; ranitidine (Zantac), nizatidine (Axid), and famotidine (Pepcid) soon followed. These medications mostly affect meal-induced acid production but work poorly in between meals. Both prescription and over-the-counter (OTC) forms are available.

H2 blockers are less expensive, less potent, shorter-acting acid suppressors than the next generation to come along: the proton-pump inhibitors, or PPIs. Proton-pump inhibitors are the most potent acid-blocking drugs available. Omeprazole (Prilosec) was the first one to come on the market, in 1989. Five other PPIs are now sold in the United States: dexlansoprazole (Dexilant), esomeprazole (Nexium), lansoprazole (Prevacid), rabeprazole (Aciphex), and pantoprazole (Protonix). In 2009, approximately 21 million people filled at least one PPI prescription. About 113 million prescriptions for them are filled globally each year. More recently, these powerful medications have become available over the counter and are vigorously promoted by manufacturers. (Think of television ads for Nexium, the "purple pill.") Several years ago the total cost expenditure on PPIs was more than $13 billion. I consider a great deal of that cost to be attributed to inappropriate use of these drugs.

Blocking acid is a necessary aspect of treating certain medical conditions. PPIs are used to heal stomach and intestinal ulcers, treat inflammation and erosions in the esophagus from reflux, prevent Barrett's esophagus (a precancerous condition), prevent ulcers in critically ill patients in intensive care units, and help eradicate *Helicobacter pylori,* an organism that causes many upper gastrointestinal (GI) problems. PPIs have been shown to be superior to H2 blockers in healing gastric and intestinal ulcers and in the treatment of *H. pylori*. For most acute medical conditions, therapy with drugs of either class should not exceed 90 days. (Barrett's esophagus and severe inflammation in the esophagus may require longer treatment.)

For mild cases of GERD and indigestion, the two classes of medication are equally effective, but they should be considered short-term solutions only. When people take them regularly, they can cause real trouble.

Here are the stories of two patients.

Elena, a sixty-five-year-old woman with osteoarthritis, had been prescribed daily naproxen (Aleve) for joint pain. After three months on the drug, she developed dark, black stools and felt light-headed. During an emergency room visit, she was found to have a gastrointestinal bleed from an ulcer in her stomach. She was admitted to the hospital, where the doctors took her off the naproxen, gave her 40 milligrams via IV of the proton-pump inhibitor pantoprazole twice a day, and performed an endoscopy. The bleeding stopped, and she was discharged with a prescription for oral pantoprazole, 40 milligrams twice daily with six refills.

Six months later, an upper respiratory tract infection brought Elena back to the doctor's office, where she was prescribed the antibiotic amoxicillin. After three days on it, she developed severe diarrhea and was diagnosed with *Clostridium difficile (C. diff)* colitis. Her doctor told her that the PPI had made her more susceptible to this serious infection, which required more aggressive antibiotic therapy, and that she would be at higher risk for recurrence of *C. diff* if she continued it.

John, age fifty-two, asked his new primary care provider for a refill of the omeprazole he had been faithfully taking for the past five years following a diagnosis of GERD. Back then, he had experienced gradually worsening heartburn as well as frequent belching. His then primary care doctor referred him to a gastroenterologist, who performed an endoscopy that showed only mild inflammation of the lower esophagus. Neither doctor took a dietary history from John or inquired about other aspects of his lifestyle. He was started on omeprazole, which eliminated the heartburn, although whenever he tried to stop taking the medication, his symptoms returned with a vengeance. He was disappointed to be so dependent on drug therapy, but the gastroenterologist had assured him that omeprazole was safe, and besides, what else could he do?

Then his wife showed him an article about long-term consequences of suppressing stomach acid, including infection and reduced absorption of important nutrients. He decided to stop the omeprazole cold turkey and, just as in the past, his heartburn returned within days, worse than ever. He had recently been switched to a new primary care physician but had yet to meet with her. He telephoned her to request a refill of his prescription, but the doctor insisted that she have the chance to evaluate him first. At their meeting, he described what happened when he stopped taking the medication, expecting that this would indicate the need for continued, possibly lifelong, treatment with a PPI.

The doctor, however, explained the phenomenon of rebound acid hypersecretion—a worsening of heartburn symptoms that commonly occurs after sudden cessation of PPI use. This can last months, she said, but alone did not mean he would need to stay on the drug. In addition, she went over the long list of possible side effects of PPIs, and expressed her opinion that he should stop taking them. She suggested weaning off the medication very slowly, cutting the dose according to a schedule she gave him. She told him also that if he experienced significant discomfort on a lower dose, he should not hesitate to go back up to the previous amount for a week or so, then try again to cut it. And she gave him handouts detailing dietary changes he should strongly consider, such as reducing caffeine and alcohol intake, as well as stress-management techniques, including breath work, that over time could help soothe the irritated lining of his esophagus. She even mentioned natural remedies that might help in a pinch.

John was skeptical of her approach, convinced that without the PPI, his heartburn would never go away. But the doctor assured him that he could successfully discontinue the medicine if he followed the schedule. That was all the motivation he needed to commit to the recommended changes. It wasn't easy for John; over the next few months, as he gradually decreased the dose of omeprazole, the pain at times made him very uncomfortable. During these episodes he questioned his doctor's guidance, but she encouraged him to stick with it. After six months, he was completely off the PPI and symptom-free. His whole family adopted the satisfying eating plan he was on, and he continued to practice the stress-management techniques he had learned. At a follow-up appointment, John told his doctor that he had never felt better.

HOW H2 BLOCKERS WORK

H2 blockers inhibit the action of the regulatory substance histamine on the acid-secreting cells in the stomach, decreasing their production of acid. The body develops tolerance to these drugs over time, lessening their effectiveness. H2 blockers work more rapidly than PPIs (within thirty minutes) and have a shorter duration of action (no more than twelve hours). They can be used as needed to control symptoms, not just as maintenance therapy, and work best at blocking surges in stomach acid in response to eating. These drugs are meant to be taken thirty minutes before meals, and no more than twice a day.

How PPIs Work

PPIs block the last stage in gastric acid production—the operation of the "proton pump" in acid-secreting cells. This mechanism takes potassium ions from inside the stomach and exchanges them for acidic hydrogen ions. PPIs are potent agents, decreasing gastric acid secretion by up to 99 percent. And because they bind irreversibly to and deactivate the proton pump, the effect of a single daily dose lasts almost a full twenty-four hours. Intake of food or other antacids at the same time decreases the efficacy of PPIs, as these medications require an acidic environment to be activated. Thus they should be taken on an empty stomach thirty minutes prior to a meal to obtain maximum benefit. Maximal effects occur after five to seven days of regular use; taking them intermittently may not suppress acid sufficiently to produce satisfactory clinical results.

THE PROBLEMS WITH H2 BLOCKERS AND PPIs

In the short term, H2 blockers may cause constipation, diarrhea, nausea, or vomiting. They may also affect the central nervous system, causing confusion, lethargy, headaches, and dizziness, especially in elderly patients and those with kidney or liver dysfunction. Cimetidine appears to cause more central nervous system side effects than the other three H2 blockers.

Headaches, nausea, abdominal pain, diarrhea, skin rashes, dizziness, weakness, and constipation are the most commonly reported short-term side effects of PPIs.

Short-term use of these medications is generally well tolerated. However, with both H2 blockers and PPIs so widely available, many consumers take them casually with little or no awareness of their long-term risks.

Dependence

The most serious risk of long-term PPI therapy is dependence—a striking example of the homeostatic trap that ensnares patients who use suppressive medications over the long term. The body reacts to suppression of acid production in the stomach by trying to make more of it. As soon as the drugs are stopped or the dosage reduced, acid secretion increases, with consequent worsening of symptoms. This common reaction is known as *rebound acid hypersecretion* and is defined as an increase in gastric acid secretion above levels prior to starting therapy. Symptoms of heartburn, indigestion, and dyspepsia (burping up of gas and stomach juices) develop within two weeks of PPI cessation. Patients (and their doctors) may falsely believe that these symptoms argue for further therapy with PPIs when, in fact, they are a withdrawal reaction associated with dependence on the medication. In one study, healthy individuals without heartburn, reflux, or acid indigestion were given 40 milligrams of esomeprazole daily for eight weeks; upon cessation, most of them experienced acid-related symptoms. In other words, over time, these drugs can cause the very problem they are meant to treat.

Dependence on PPIs is very stubborn. Most people affected by it have great difficulty getting off these drugs. Integrative medicine practitioners recommend weaning off them slowly while instituting the lifestyle measures and other therapies described on page 77.

Disruption of the Microbiome

Altering the acidity of the stomach disrupts the normal gut microbiome — the population of microorganisms living in the lower GI tract that are necessary for normal digestion and GI function and strongly influence all aspects of health. Long-term use of acid-suppressing drugs can inhibit normal, beneficial organisms, while encouraging overgrowth of harmful bacteria.

Pneumonia

Reduced acid diminishes the stomach's ability to maintain a sterile environment free of bacteria, viruses, and yeast. Some studies suggest there may be a higher rate of pneumonia in those taking H2s and PPIs due to silent reflux and aspiration of gastric contents into the lungs.

GI Infections

Reduced gastric acidity can promote bacterial overgrowth in the small intestine, making patients more vulnerable to colonization and illness caused by pathogens like *C. diff*. Rates and recurrences of *C. diff* infection are higher than average in patients on PPI therapy. They are also elevated, but less so, in those on H2 blockers. People with low stomach acid are more susceptible to cholera and certain infections contracted by eating raw shellfish.

Micronutrient Deficiency

Gastric acid is important for breaking down and digesting food and releasing nutrients and vitamins. Problems with iron and B_{12} absorption are typically mild and easily corrected with oral supplementation, but magnesium deficiency may have more serious consequences, including heart arrhythmias and seizures. In March 2011 the FDA issued a safety warning regarding this risk. It advised doctors to check serum magnesium levels prior to starting on a PPI and monitor them periodically for the duration of the therapy.

Poor Absorption of Calcium and Impaired Bone Health

PPI therapy can block calcium absorption, leading to osteoporosis and fractures. To prevent these problems the FDA recommends using the lowest effective dose for the shortest duration of time as well as supplementing with calcium and vitamin D.

Cardiac Disease

A recent study brought to light the possibility of an increased risk of heart attack in patients using PPIs long term (but no such risk in those on H2 blockers). The risk was shown to be in the general population and not just among patients who were at high risk or had a history of cardiac disease. The reason is not clear but may involve adverse effects on blood vessels.

Kidney Disease

Evidence suggests an association between PPI use, kidney inflammation, and increased risk of chronic kidney disease (CKD). As noted earlier, PPIs reduce absorption of magnesium. They also appear to induce immune-mediated kidney damage. Both may contribute to the development of CKD. The author of one recent study on this risk writes, "The results emphasize the importance of limiting PPI use to only when it is medically necessary, and also limiting the duration of use to the shortest duration possible."

Dementia

A study examining the use of PPIs in people age seventy-five and older showed that taking the medication was associated with a 44 percent increased risk of dementia. The finding is not definitive, but it raises serious concerns about the use of PPIs in the elderly.

Medication Interactions

H2 blockers have multiple interactions with other medications, including antibiotics, antivirals, and anticoagulants. Before starting on one of them, patients should check with their doctor or pharmacist to make certain there are no interactions of concern.

Integrative Medicine Approaches to Managing GERD

Despite their shortcomings and the many serious consequences of long-term use, PPIs and H2 blockers are commonly given as first-line treatments for acid reflux, dyspepsia, and heartburn. Once started on PPIs or H2 blockers, many people continue to take them indefinitely. Too often doctors prescribe them without inquiring into the dietary habits, stress levels, and other aspects of patients' lives known to affect GI function. And too often patients take OTC forms of these drugs without giving any thought to managing their symptoms in other, safer ways, such as those described below.

Dietary Modification

Examining and changing dietary habits should be a primary approach to managing GERD.

The lower esophageal sphincter (LES) keeps acidic gastric contents within the stomach and out of the esophagus. It is normal for some amount of stomach acid to reflux into the lower esophagus with transient relaxation of the LES. In people with GERD, periods of relaxation are more prolonged and frequent. A common cause of this is distension of the stomach from overeating. High intra-abdominal pressure associated with obesity also predisposes to reflux, leading to heartburn, GERD, and esophagitis. (Waist size has a direct correlation to the risk of developing reflux esophagitis and to its severity and attendant risk of developing cancer. Weight loss can significantly help with these symptoms and prevent long-term complications.)

These dietary strategies are worth trying: consuming frequent small meals, avoiding high-fat meals, and limiting spicy and acidic foods—such as citrus and tomatoes—as well as coffee (caffeinated and decaffeinated) and other caffeinated drinks, chocolate, alcohol, carbonated beverages, onions, and garlic. An upright position should be maintained for at least three hours after eating to allow food to digest and empty from the stomach. Elevating the head of the bed at night and sleeping on the left side have been shown to benefit patients with nighttime reflux symptoms.

Finally, there is some literature to support that food allergies may be a contributor to GERD symptoms, and even that PPIs may promote the development of food allergies by disrupting the gut microbiome. Cow's milk allergy in children is a well-known cause of GERD that does not respond to PPI therapy. Following a gluten-free diet improves symptoms of GERD in those with celiac disease.

Other Lifestyle Measures

Smoking is a potent relaxer of the LES. Smoking cessation reduces acid reflux and decreases the risk of gastritis.

Avoiding or limiting nonsteroidal anti-inflammatory drugs (NSAIDs, such as ibuprofen, aspirin, and naproxen) is important; used frequently, they strongly irritate the lining of the stomach and increase the risk of bleeding.

Stress is a notorious trigger for heartburn. A prominent

symptom of anxiety is the feeling of a knot or "butter-flies" in the stomach, a familiar example of the connection between that organ and emotions. A recent study of GERD patients showed that feeling stressed was the most common lifestyle factor correlated with the disorder, present in 45.6 percent of 12,653 patients surveyed. Up to 50 percent of first responders involved in the 9/11 attacks in New York City suffered from post-traumatic stress disorder (PTSD), with 70 percent of them having chronic reflux-related symptoms.

In states of chronic stress and anxiety, the body's gut-brain hormonal regulation is disrupted. As part of the flight-or-flight response, heightened sympathetic nervous system activity freezes stomach motility and relaxes the LES, increasing the possibility of reflux. Under stress there is also a breakdown of the integrity of cells in the lining of the stomach, making it more vulnerable to irritation by acid and digestive enzymes.

There are many practices to consider for neutralizing the harmful effects of stress on the body and mind: tai chi, yoga, meditation, hypnotherapy, breath work, and more.

Coating Agents

Sucralfate (Carafate) is a prescription medication that protects the gut lining, without any of the long-term adverse effects of H2 blockers and PPIs. It coats ulcers and erosions as well as "cracks," protecting tissues from the caustic effects of acid and digestive enzymes. It can actually heal erosions and ulcers, something the acid-suppressive drugs cannot do.

Natural products that strengthen the protective mucous lining of the stomach and esophagus include slippery elm *(Ulmus fulva)* powder or lozenges and deglycyrrhizinated licorice (DGL) powder or chewable tablets to be taken before meals and at bedtime.

Approximately 60 percent of patients who experience GERD have a hiatal hernia—a protrusion of part of the stomach into the chest cavity. This impairs the ability of the LES to prevent acid reflux and also creates a pocket that retains irritating gastric juices; these tend to back up into the esophagus. OTC coating medications, like Gaviscon, are available for the problem. They contain alginate (made from brown algae) and bicarbonate, which together coat the stomach lining and form a barrier against reflux from the pocket. A recent study has shown these agents to be as effective as PPIs for management of GERD associated with hiatal hernia.

Protecting the lining of the stomach and esophagus from acid irritation versus suppressing acid production with powerful drugs illustrates the difference between Eastern and Western medical philosophy. A wise practitioner of modern Chinese medicine once told me that his goal was "to dispel evil and support the good." Western medicine focuses mostly on dispelling evil, especially by using drugs to oppose or destroy what it sees as causes of disease: antibiotics against harmful bacteria, for example, and suppressive drugs to block acid secretion in the stomach. Eastern medicine directs much more attention to supporting the good—that is, protecting and enhancing the body's natural defenses. Integrative medicine uses both approaches. In the case of GERD, making the lining of the gut more resistant to the potentially irritating effects of acid may be as important as trying to make acid go away—or even more so.

Antacids

Simple antacids, like calcium carbonate, provide fast and effective short-term relief of heartburn and symptoms of GERD. They also promote esophageal motility to clear acid from that organ. Used frequently, they may cause constipation, which can be mitigated by taking supplemental magnesium. I recommend avoiding aluminum-containing antacids (like Maalox and Mylanta), because of possible harmful effects of that element.

Other Natural Products

Many herbal therapies are available for the treatment of GI disorders. Ginger has been shown in numerous studies to help with nausea, vomiting, and GI upset. When consumed in the form of capsules containing powdered root, ginger promotes gastric motility. Two to three teaspoons of apple cider vinegar mixed in 8 ounces of water may help relieve acid reflux by mechanisms that are not yet fully understood. Chamomile tea can help soothe stomach inflammation. (Avoid peppermint tea, often used for simple indigestion; it worsens GERD by relaxing the LES.) Aloe juice, a popular home remedy to soothe inflamed and irritated skin, can also soothe internal inflammation. A half cup of the juice twice a day is the recommended dose. D-limonene, derived from the rind of lemons, helps promote healthy gastric motility and prevent reflux; dosage is 1000 milligrams once every other day for a total of ten doses, then as needed.

A few studies have shown benefit in 6 milligrams of melatonin taken at bedtime. Melatonin is a safe and effective remedy for insomnia. Poor sleep promotes GERD, and GERD interferes with sleep. Melatonin is also a weak blocker of stomach acid and may increase LES tone; one study showed it to be as effective as a PPI when used in combination with other supplements, such as DGL.

BOTTOM LINE

GERD is a complex problem marked by decreased resilience of the GI tract to deal with external and internal stressors. Heartburn is a warning sign of disturbed GI function that should prompt us to identify and change the habits responsible for it. A pill that blocks stomach acid will make symptoms of GERD disappear as if by magic but cannot address its root causes. Over time, the pill will become less effective, create dependence, and increase risks of more serious problems. It is best to use H2 blockers and PPIs for short-term therapy and for longer-term management only of relatively rare, very severe conditions. Addressing the root causes of GERD with lifestyle changes and safe and effective alternative remedies is a much better approach.

4

Antihistamines

Allergies had been part of Amit's life since childhood—beginning with seasonal symptoms: watery and itchy eyes, runny nose, nasal congestion, and uncontrollable sneezing fits. Antihistamines managed these symptoms, but by the time Amit turned thirty-five, his allergies were present year-round, and the drugs had become less effective. Worse were the unacceptable side effects. Not only did he feel like he was "operating in a cloud" while on them, but his wife noticed a change in his mood: he was more volatile and argumentative. Amit's doctor tried him on several "non-sedating" antihistamines, but they failed to control his symptoms. He twice tried desensitization (allergy shots) but got no benefit and once nearly died from a severe reaction (anaphylaxis). Although nasal corticosteroid sprays helped marginally, his nose continued to run. Doses of prednisone and other oral steroids worked for Amit but kept him up all night and made him so moody that co-workers avoided him.

By the time he was fifty-five years old, he had tried just about every prescription therapy available, each with drawbacks. His dependable older antihistamines now caused a new symptom that was shocking—pain and difficulty emptying his bladder, prompting one panicky visit to an emergency room.

It was at this point that Amit became fearful of drugs and sought a more integrative approach. He saw a practitioner who recommended fundamental changes in Amit's lifestyle: an anti-inflammatory diet* along with meditation and breath control to relax. Amit learned about the effectiveness of freeze-dried stinging nettle leaves for hay fever, and found that two capsules totally eliminated his itching and sneezing, although he had to repeat the dose as often as every four hours during the day. He experienced no side effects at all from this herbal remedy.

Through all the years of relying on suppressive medication, his symptoms had persisted and gotten worse. After two seasons of this alternative regimen, his hay fever subsided and eventually disappeared.

---

* For details of the anti-inflammatory diet, see Andrew Weil, *Healthy Aging* (New York: Knopf, 2005), chapter 9, pp. 140–160. Also: http://www.drweil.com/drw/u/ART02012/anti-inflammatory-diet.

ALLERGIC REACTIONS

Allergies have plagued us throughout history; records from ancient Egypt describe them. The development of an immune system was a major milestone in evolution that helped ensure our survival, but with it came complications.

It has been proposed that allergies represent the immune system "going awry"; however, this may not be the case. Many believe that allergic reactions originally served to eradicate parasites, which were much more of a problem before we lived in clean environments, seriously threatening human health. The allergies that cause us trouble today may be evolutionary remnants of this parasitic defense system, now inappropriately redirected against harmless substances in the environment, such as pollen. An alternative theory is that allergic reactions evolved to help rid the body of, or protect it from, toxins. Some evidence for this is the fact that most allergy symptoms serve to expel irritants from the body—whether through sneezing, a runny nose, watery eyes, or, in the case of food allergies, diarrhea.

Hay fever, or allergic rhinitis, affects about 8 percent of adults in the United States and is responsible for more than 11 million visits to physician offices annually. We try to deal with allergens as we deal with many conflicts in life: by avoidance. Unfortunately, pollens from grasses and trees are wind-borne and hard to avoid.

How Antihistamines Work

The allergic reaction releases chemicals that are stored inside a specialized immune cell called the mast cell. The mast cell is like a time bomb, waiting for an allergen to set it off. After activation, it breaks open, rapidly releasing its store of potent chemical messengers, histamine among them. Once histamine gets into the bloodstream, it binds to special receptors in blood vessels, smooth muscle, and elsewhere, causing such allergic symptoms as itching, flushing, headache, runny nose, and occasionally shortness of breath and wheezing.

Antihistamine drugs bind to the same receptors and block these symptoms — but only if they get there first. To do the most good, they have to be used prior to the start of the reaction. Once the reaction has started, taking an antihistamine will still be useful but not as effective as a prophylactic dose.

Common Uses for Antihistamines

Most commonly, antihistamines are used for relief of seasonal or perennial nasal and ocular allergies — the stuffiness, runny nose, and itchy and watery eye symptoms that are the hallmark of an allergy attack. Some people use these drugs in an attempt to treat similar symptoms that occur with a common cold or the flu (see chapter 5), but their benefit here is minimal.

There are, however, other common indications for antihistamines. Arguably, their most important use is in the treatment of anaphylaxis, the most dangerous allergic reaction. People with severe allergies to certain foods, insects, or drugs can develop this life-threatening reaction, marked by a sudden drop in blood pressure, airway closure, and consequent breathing difficulties. Prompt treatment is necessary to prevent death — with potent drugs such as epinephrine (adrenalin) and corticosteroids, along with aggressive intravenous hydration. Antihistamines, given in large doses intravenously, can also help arrest the reaction and save a life.

Urticaria — hives — can be caused by contact with a provocative trigger (such as poison ivy), ingestion of a specific food, or stress, or it can occur for no apparent reason. Hives can erupt all over the body, usually accompanied by severe itching (pruritus). Antihistamines offer some level of relief from the incessant itch, while at the same time facilitating needed sleep.

One reason to use antihistamines is supported more by advertising than by research. Many people with insomnia, and without access to the more expensive (and harmful) prescription sleep drugs, have been persuaded to use over-the-counter (OTC) products like Simply Sleep, Unisom, Tylenol PM, and others that contain the antihistamine diphenhydramine (Benadryl) in various doses. True, this compound causes drowsiness, but is the sleep quality the same as that of natural sleep? Most experts say no; overall sleep quality after taking Benadryl is usually not very good. In addition, most users suffer side effects of dry mouth, urinary retention, and a high frequency of next-day sluggishness and mental clouding.

THE PROBLEMS WITH ANTIHISTAMINES

Antihistamines are among the oldest drugs still in use, discovered in 1937 by Daniel Bovet, who later won a Nobel Prize for his work. Among the most commonly sold OTC medications in the United States are cough-cold and allergy remedies, many of which are, or include, antihistamines. The fact that they are available without a prescription leads many people to believe that they are perfectly safe, which is simply not true. Many of their adverse effects become apparent only after many years of use.

The first antihistamines have a long track record, and most of their adverse effects are known. They include diphenhydramine (Benadryl), chlorpheniramine (Chlor-Trimeton), clemastine (Tavist), and others. By nature of their chemical structure, these drugs readily cross the blood-brain barrier, affecting the central nervous system. First-generation antihistamines cause significant sedation. In fact, they can impair driving ability as much as or more than alcohol. The impairment can be subtle: prior to falling asleep on antihistamines, there is a drowsy period with mental fogginess and a decline in thought processes that may not be apparent to the patient.

The search for less sedating (incorrectly termed "non-sedating") antihistamines led to the discovery of a second generation of drugs. The first of these, terfenadine (Seldane), was released in 1985 to great fanfare and an advertising blitz. Within a few years, serious heart arrhythmias were reported, especially when the drug was taken with certain antibiotics. By the time Seldane was removed from the market, it was blamed for eight deaths—in people who were just trying to stop sneezing. Other drugs in this class include fexofenadine (Allegra), loratadine (Claritin), and cetirizine (Zyrtec). While a smaller amount of these medications crosses the blood-brain barrier, they still cause drowsiness, prompting the warning to "be careful when driving a motor vehicle or operating machinery." Unfortunately, many users continue to drive under their influence—a potential public health hazard. In elderly patients, the risks are elevated, with potential adverse effects of next-day sedation, dizziness, and falls.

Both first- and second-generation antihistamines can affect mood and cognitive function, causing or worsening depression and interfering with thinking and concentration. Anyone struggling with depression should avoid them.

And more ominous adverse effects have been attributed to these popular drugs. A recent study of more than three thousand men and women over the age of sixty-five revealed a link between long-term use of anticholinergic medications, including Benadryl and other first-generation antihistamines, and the risk of dementia. (Anticholinergic drugs block the action of acetylcholine, a neurotransmitter in the brain, and include the tricyclic antidepressants, discussed in chapter 9, as well as the older antihistamines.) Taking such medications for the equivalent of three years or more increased the risk of developing dementia by 54 percent. Other notable anticholinergic effects that have been seen with first-generation antihistamines are low blood pressure, delirium, and behavioral changes. In men, particularly those with an enlarged prostate gland, these drugs can cause urinary retention — both acute and chronic. Rarely, this can lead to severe bladder and kidney dysfunction.

Other adverse effects attributed to antihistamines have been proposed but are still under investigation. They are, however, concerning. There is a body of evidence linking antihistamine use with the development of brain tumors, especially gliomas. Gliomas are the most common primary malignant brain tumors, and few risk factors for them have been identified. However, several studies show that people who report regular long-term use of antihistamines are nearly three times as likely as non-users to develop these tumors, regardless of asthma/allergy history. These data are more interesting in view of the fact that an inverse relationship between allergies and glioma is one of the most consistent associations in the brain tumor literature. I wonder if allergies have a protective effect of some sort that is negated by antihistamines.

Drug therapy for allergies, taken as a whole and including OTC medications, costs more than $6 billion per year. An individual taking a second-generation antihistamine could spend anywhere from $8 to more than $200 per month.

Integrative Medicine Approaches to Managing Allergic Conditions

There are many effective methods for managing allergies that do not rely on antihistamines. One of the more obvious is avoidance — reducing contact with allergens by using common-sense strategies. High-efficiency particulate air (HEPA) filters, which remove particles from the air by forcing it through screens with microscopic

pores, work well for lighter-weight allergens like pet dan-
der and not so well for heavier ones like most pollen
particles.

Frequent nasal irrigation with a warm saline solution (¼ teaspoon salt to 1 cup distilled water) will flush
allergenic particles from the lining tissue of the nose. A
neti pot is often employed for this purpose. This device
resembles an Aladdin's lamp made of ceramic, glass, or
plastic and is easy to use, although the practice may
take some getting used to. Pour sterile saline into the
neti pot. Then, standing over a sink with your head
tilted about 45 degrees to one side, place the spout into
the higher nostril and slowly pour the solution into
your nose. Spit out any liquid that enters your mouth.
Once the neti pot is empty, gently blow your nose, tilt
your head the opposite way, and repeat the process with
the other nostril.

Many supplements and botanicals have proven value
in controlling allergic rhinitis. Stinging nettle *(Urtica
dioica)* is one of the best natural remedies. It is best
taken in freeze-dried form in capsules. In a randomized, double-blind study of nearly one hundred patients,
57 percent rated nettle effective in relieving allergic rhinitis symptoms, and 48 percent said it equaled or sur-
passed the effectiveness of previously used allergy
medications. It is a symptomatic treatment, not a preventive one; the usual dose is one or two capsules every
two to four hours as needed.

Butterbur *(Petasites hybridus)* has been used for decades to treat allergies as well as asthma and migraine headaches and is one of the few botanicals to go head-to-head with a drug in a clinical trial. A study of 132 people with hay fever found that an extract of this herb was as effective as cetirizine (Zyrtec) with fewer side effects; butterbur was also much less sedating than the pharmaceutical product. The study lasted only two weeks and required four to five doses of the herb daily, but results were promising.

Bioflavonoids are compounds that give many vegetables and fruits their bright colors. They also have remarkable activity in allergic diseases — they actually *prevent* mast cells from "exploding" and releasing histamine. Like antihistamines, these compounds work best when taken in advance of an allergen exposure; as stated above, preventing histamine release is always preferable to trying to mitigate its effects once it gets into the bloodstream. Unlike antihistamines, bioflavonoids have few side effects. Some, like quercetin and fisetin, are available in supplement form. (Due to poor bioavailability, quercetin is often combined with bromelain — an enzyme found in pineapple — or vitamin C to improve oral absorption.) Because effects of bioflavonoids are not long lasting, they must be taken every four to six hours, but they work very well for many patients. Cromolyn, a bioflavonoid-related mast-cell stabilizer, is available in nasal sprays (like NasalCrom) and in nebulizers (for allergic asthma). I consider it safe and effective.

Mind-body interventions have been shown to modify allergic responses. In a controlled setting, allergic individuals received skin tests to assess their reactivity to allergens after viewing either a documentary dealing with the weather or a humorous movie. In those who watched the humorous film, skin test reactivity decreased significantly, demonstrating that emotions can powerfully mitigate the effects of allergen exposure. This supports the connection between the immune system and emotions, the subject of a field of study known as psychoneuroimmunology. You can take advantage of this connection with such interventions as clinical hypnotherapy, which can reduce allergic responsiveness in many people.

Most discussions of the impact of diet on allergies are limited to food allergies, but what you eat can also affect your body's reactions to airborne allergens. The body activates similar inflammatory pathways for many diverse triggers, including infection and trauma. Allergic reactions are simply inflammatory reactions with a specific allergen as the inciting catalyst. Specialized cells of the immune system produce compounds — inflammatory mediators — to contain the infection or extent of injury. Other immune cells migrate to the site of the problem to act as reinforcements. Following an anti-inflammatory diet reduces allergic reactivity by inhibiting synthesis of the inflammatory mediators. Simply adding omega-3 fats to the diet, in the form of fatty fish or fish oil supplements, can accomplish this in many people.

BOTTOM LINE

Antihistamines can save lives in the case of anaphylaxis and other severe allergic reactions. That is their greatest value. People with allergic rhinitis and others who suffer from common allergy symptoms would be wise not to rely on antihistamines but instead to try natural remedies and lifestyle changes, including dietary changes and stress management, to control symptoms. Those approaches can result in reduced allergic responsiveness and even complete disappearance of allergies. I do not see this happen in people who rely on antihistamines to suppress allergic symptoms. Like other long-term suppressive medications, they tend to perpetuate the problem they are meant to treat.

5

Medications for the Common Cold and the Flu

Anna, a forty-six-year-old woman, came to her neighborhood urgent care clinic complaining of cough, sneezing, runny nose, and sinus discomfort since the previous day. Upon signing in, she requested a prescription antibiotic, saying that she needed to get better quickly to attend an important business meeting later in the week. Medical evaluation suggested that she was experiencing the early stages of the common cold. The doctor told Anna she had contracted a viral upper respiratory infection, that she should get better within a week, and that antibiotics are not indicated for viral disorders. Anna expressed both surprise and dismay. She repeated her request for the antibiotic, saying that she knew her body and that she had always responded best in these circumstances when taking one. The physician again denied the request, adding that she should also avoid most over-the-counter (OTC) cold and cough medications because they offered little benefit and in some instances could be harmful. He recommended general supportive measures, especially plenty of rest. The patient said she understood, and they parted cordially.

Three days later the patient and doctor met again. This time Anna had a red rash all over her body except on her hands and feet, watery bowel movements, insomnia, and itching in her "private parts" associated with a white discharge. She reported that she had been very disappointed not to have received an antibiotic during her previous visit and had gone directly to another clinic where she had gotten a prescription for one. Along with that, she had also been taking two OTC cold remedies to help manage the runny nose and congestion. Her cold symptoms were now almost gone, which she attributed to the antibiotic, but the new problems were worse. She was experiencing well-known adverse effects associated with antibiotic therapy: allergic reaction, vaginal yeast infection, and diarrhea from disruption of gut flora. Her difficulty sleeping was likely due to the OTC cold products, both of which contained chemical stimulants. She was advised to stop the antibiotic and cold remedies immediately, prescribed appropriate antifungal therapy, and told to take a probiotic to help rebalance her microbiome. The doctor predicted she would be feeling better within a day or two, but cautioned that she should seek prompt medical attention if she developed shortness of breath, worsening diarrhea, fever, or abdominal pain. The latter symptoms could indicate infection with *Clostridium difficile,* a potentially dangerous condition often resulting from antibiotic therapy.

I hear stories like this all the time and believe that similar cases play out in doctors' offices around the world. Colds are a nuisance, and we have been conditioned to believe that we have to take something to help us get over them. Colds are also the most common acute human illness. Most adults experience two to three of them annually; children fare worse, getting four to twelve colds each year. Generally considered benign, colds typically resolve within a few days without the need for specific treatment, although some symptoms may persist for up to two weeks. Nonetheless, colds are associated with an enormous economic burden, including more than $3 billion spent on OTC cough and cold remedies, more than $7 billion related to physician visits, and approximately $20 billion associated with lost work and school days.

The flu is also costly and is not at all benign. Many

people with bad colds think they have the flu, but influenza is caused by a different virus, one that attacks the lower respiratory system and is associated with serious complications that can be fatal. According to World Health Organization estimates, between three and five million cases of flu-related illness occur annually, as well as 250,000 to 500,000 flu-related deaths. In the United States, the flu leads to more than 400,000 hospitalizations and thousands of deaths each year, most involving the elderly. These statistics do not include data from influenza epidemics, such as the 2009 H1N1 flu pandemic, which was noteworthy for causing severe illness and death even in previously healthy young people.

Hundreds of different viruses cause the common cold, with rhinoviruses the chief offenders, especially during the winter. Flu season runs from October through early May, peaking in January and February. Influenza viruses mutate frequently, foiling the immune system's ability to recognize them and making it difficult to design effective vaccines. When people with colds or the flu cough or sneeze, they unwittingly release viral particles into the air that can be breathed in by others or can settle onto exposed surfaces. Viruses are able to survive on human skin and surfaces for hours and can be transmitted through touch. If the nose, mouth, or eyes are then touched, infection may occur. The best ways to reduce the risk of catching a cold or the flu are to avoid symptomatic people and wash your hands frequently and properly.

Symptoms of the common cold and the flu often overlap, but there are significant differences. Cold symptoms develop slowly, with a gradual onset of sore throat, sneezing, cough, nasal congestion, and drainage, sometimes accompanied by a general feeling of malaise. Flu has a short incubation period and is associated with rapid symptom development that may include fever, chills, fatigue, body aches, headache, cough, sore throat, and congestion. Symptoms of both the common cold and the flu mostly result from the immune system's response to infection, as it releases compounds that stimulate inflammation, dilate blood vessels, and promote mucus secretion. (Most of the more than 20 million people who died in the 1918 influenza pandemic died from drowning as their lungs filled with fluid from an exaggerated immune response to the virus.)

The Flu Vaccine

Strategies to prevent, and even to treat, both the common cold and the flu are similar, with two significant exceptions—getting the annual flu vaccine and using antiviral agents (discussed in the next section). Experts disagree about the value of flu shots. Scientists have to predict which viruses will cause influenza months before the actual flu season begins in order to produce a vaccine. Sometimes their results miss the mark. Effectiveness varies from year to year, topping out at 60 to 70 percent in a good year, when a strong match exists between the vaccine and the circulating viruses. Protection is less certain in the elderly, who may require higher doses. Vaccination is particularly important for people at high risk for flu-related complications, especially the elderly, infants and young children, those with chronic underlying heart and lung disease, and the obese.

When you get a flu shot, your body responds by producing antibodies to the strains of virus present in the vaccine. Most experts believe that vaccination provides some measure of protection. Studies suggest that it can reduce the risk of heart attack as well as flu-related pneumonia. On the other hand, reviews of data from healthy vaccinated individuals suggest a modest benefit at best and question the wisdom of widespread annual flu vaccination.

A variety of flu vaccines are available. If you opt to get a flu shot, ask for one that does not contain thimerosal, a mercury-based preservative that is being phased out. Mercury is a known neurotoxin. A list of vaccines and their thimerosal content is available from the US Food and Drug Administration (FDA).

The Problems with Cold and Flu Medicines

Overuse of Antibiotics

I must repeat that the common cold and the flu are caused by viruses. Antibiotics are active against bacteria, not viruses; thus, there is no role for antibiotic therapy in the treatment of uncomplicated colds or flu.

Nor do antibiotics have a role in preventing complications, such as sinusitis, that can develop as a result of a cold or the flu. Yet every year, tens of thousands of people with these illnesses demand prescription antibiotics from their doctors. In fact, a whopping 41 percent of all antibiotic prescriptions are directed against respiratory infections, most of them unnecessary or inappropriate. This is a big problem, as we've seen, both because antibiotics are responsible for the largest number of medication-related adverse reactions and because their misuse and overuse accelerate the development of bacterial resistance, a major threat to public health (see chapter 1). If you get a cold or the flu, do not ask your doctor for an antibiotic.

Antiviral Agents

No prescription medication yet exists that is effective for the prevention or treatment of the common cold, but prescription antiviral agents are available for flu treatment. Like the vaccine, they are of greatest benefit to those at risk for complications. Most healthy people who get the flu will be uncomfortable—sometimes *very* uncomfortable—for a few days but get better on their own, unless they have an unusually virulent strain of the virus, the kind that circulates during a world-wide influenza pandemic. Newer antivirals, termed neuraminidase inhibitors (NAIs), include zanamivir (Relenza) and oseltamivir (Tamiflu). These drugs impair the release of newly formed viral particles from infected cells. When first introduced, the NAIs were trumpeted as *the* treatment of choice for the flu. Experience suggests this was an overstatement. Studies show that NAIs shorten the duration of flu by about one day only. Alongside vaccination, they do appear to help prevent complications in those at risk, but they also have drawbacks. Zanamivir is associated with bronchospasm (wheezing) in individuals with chronic lung problems, while oseltamivir is known to cause dizziness, nausea, and vomiting. And just as bacteria have become resistant to antibiotics, the flu virus is beginning to develop resistance to NAIs, specifically to oseltamivir.

I would ask you to keep in mind that most people who contract the flu do not require medical attention or antiviral drugs, and they get better on their own.

OTC COLD AND FLU REMEDIES

It is estimated that 70 percent of cold and flu sufferers turn to OTC remedies. Most are ineffective, do not reduce the duration of illness, and are potentially dangerous, especially for children (see chapter 16). In 2008, the FDA issued a public health advisory stating that OTC cough and cold medications should not be given to infants and children under the age of two. Advisory action for all children under age eleven remains under consideration.

Many OTC cold and flu remedies contain acetaminophen (Tylenol) or nonsteroidal anti-inflammatory drugs (NSAIDs) such as ibuprofen (Advil, Motrin) (see chapter 8). These products can help reduce fever and relieve body aches when dosed appropriately. But fever is a useful response to infection; at higher body temperatures the immune system's defenses operate more efficiently. Unless fever is dangerously high (over 105°F/40.5°C), it may be wiser to make yourself comfortable with sponge baths and cool compresses than to lower fever with a drug.* Acetaminophen and NSAIDs are at best marginally effective for other cold and flu

---

* Children, adolescents, and especially infants are an exception to this statement. Any child with a fever should be evaluated by the primary care physician to determine the cause and appropriate treatment.

symptoms and can cause serious adverse effects. Some data suggest that acetaminophen may actually suppress the immune response and worsen congestion in adults, and inadvertent acetaminophen overdose can lead to liver damage.

Antihistamines (see chapter 4) are mostly used for allergies, but people often take them for cold and flu symptoms—with minimal effect. Older antihistamines, such as diphenhydramine (Benadryl), can actually make things worse because they create thicker mucus that is harder to clear. These first-generation antihistamines are also sedating, making driving and the use of heavy machinery while taking them potentially dangerous. Newer second-generation antihistamines such as fexofenadine (Allegra), loratadine (Claritin), and cetirizine (Zyrtec) are supposed to be non-sedating, but they too can make you groggy or sleepy.

Cough medicines come in two forms—antitussives containing dextromethorphan, a compound related to opioids that temporarily suppresses the cough reflex, and expectorants—often with guaifenesin, long purported to thin mucus and make it easier to clear the airways but, in fact, minimally effective. Coughing is the body's way of clearing mucus that may be compromising breathing passages. Dry coughs that are painful or debilitating, keep you up at night, or otherwise interfere with your daily activities can be effectively suppressed with dextromethorphan; productive coughs should not be suppressed.

Sometimes coughing can continue for weeks after a severe respiratory infection; the term for this is *post-viral tussive syndrome*. If dextromethorphan fails to control the cough, a prescription opioid may be necessary.

Since congestion is a symptom common to both colds and the flu, oral decongestants are another popular class of OTC remedies. Congestion results from the dilation of blood vessels in the tissue lining the airway passages. Decongestants are chemically related to epinephrine (adrenalin), a stimulant. They activate receptors that shrink blood vessels down to normal size, thereby reducing swelling and congestion. There are problems with them, however. One agent, phenylpropanolamine, was removed from the market after it was found to increase risk of death in the elderly. Marketing of another decongestant compound, pseudoephedrine, has been restricted due to its illicit use to make methamphetamine. At present, most OTC oral decongestants contain a related stimulant, phenylephrine. Side effects include anxiety, dizziness, insomnia, palpitations, and, rarely, high blood pressure.

You can spray a topical decongestant, such as oxymetazoline (Afrin), directly into the nostrils. It provides more rapid relief than oral products do but should be used for only a short period of time, perhaps one to three days. With longer use, effectiveness wanes and you find yourself spraying it into your nose more frequently to manage rebound congestion (known as rhinitis medicamentosa). This represents the body's homeostatic reaction to the drug: nasal congestion worsens and persists. Continual use of topical decongestants makes for a vicious cycle of drug dependence.

Since all decongestants are stimulants, caution is recommended for people with poorly controlled hypertension, irregular heart rhythms, heart disease, or glaucoma. These medications can also impair bladder muscle activity, leading to urinary retention. Those with known urinary dysfunction, as well as men with an enlarged prostate gland, should avoid them.

Many OTC cold and cough remedies combine pain relievers, cough suppressants, decongestants, and antihistamines. If you plan to use them, be sure to read the labels carefully—doubling up on certain compounds puts you at greater risk for toxic side effects. Some evidence suggests that these products may actually prolong illness by giving people the sense that they are treating the problem and can go about their business instead of resting to conserve energy.

INTEGRATIVE MEDICINE APPROACHES TO TREATING COLDS AND THE FLU

Herbal Remedies and Supplements

A variety of herbs and supplements can be used for the management of colds and the flu. Andrographis

(Andrographis paniculata), an herb commonly used in traditional Indian medicine (Ayurveda), has been shown to reduce symptoms both alone and when combined with another herb, eleuthero *(Eleutherococcus senticosus).* Astragalus *(Astragalus membranaceus),* obtained from the root of a plant in the pea family, has been used for centuries in China to ward off respiratory infections. I recommend it preventively throughout cold and flu season, especially for people who tend to catch "everything going around." I take it myself when I fly or am exposed to people who are coughing and sneezing. Astragalus is nontoxic and can be taken indefinitely. Echinacea *(Echinacea angustifolia, purpurea,* or *pallida)* can help the immune system fight infection, but results of studies examining its effects on the common cold have been mixed. Standardized extracts that contain both *E. purpurea* and *E. angustifolia* seem to be most effective, especially in adults. Elderberry *(Sambucus nigra)* has both anti-inflammatory and antiviral properties, and studies suggest it can significantly reduce the duration of flu symptoms; it is available in syrups and lozenges. In addition to its use in the kitchen, garlic *(Allium sativum)* is a powerful therapeutic herb with immune-stimulating properties as well as antiviral and antibacterial effects. I eat a small amount of raw garlic at the first sign of a cold, chopping a few cloves into my food. Products made from the African geranium *(Pelargonium sidoides)* may reduce the

severity and duration of a cold. The homeopathic remedy Oscillococcinum, made from duck liver and heart, is promoted for treatment of the flu, but supportive evidence is weak. Probiotics may protect against fever, cough, and runny nose in children, but the data are less compelling for adults.

Most studies conclude that prophylactic vitamin C (200 to 500 milligrams daily, with larger doses supported in some studies) may help prevent the common cold, or at least reduce the severity and duration of symptoms. It seems most effective for those who are vitamin C deficient. Epidemiologic data suggest a correlation between vitamin D levels and the incidence of upper respiratory tract infections, including the flu. (Blood levels of vitamin D are lowest during winter months, when the incidence of colds and the flu is highest.) Research findings are mixed, but vitamin D supplementation may help prevent colds and flu in those with low levels. Zinc deficiency impairs immune system function, and studies using zinc sulfate, acetate, and gluconate against the common cold suggest a trend toward benefit if taken within the first twenty-four hours, although overall the evidence is weak. Adverse effects, such as nausea, are more common with lozenges than with syrups or tablets. Intranasal zinc may result in permanent damage to an individual's sense of smell.

Lifestyle Modifications

Smokers are at increased risk for contracting respiratory tract infections and can reduce that risk by quitting. Chronic stress, lack of social support, and depression can all interfere with immune function, increasing risk of infection. Stress management practices and social engagement can be protective as well as enjoyable. Mindfulness meditation has been shown to reduce the incidence, severity, and duration of cold symptoms, as has moderate exercise. Excessive exercise, however, such as vigorous running, may temporarily increase the risk of infection. Adequate sleep is critically important in supporting optimal immune system function. If you get fewer than six hours of sleep a night, you are more likely to get a cold because the sleep-deprived body produces fewer of the natural killer cells it needs to destroy virus-infected cells. Aim for at least seven hours of sleep each night.

Bottom Line

Colds and the flu are common, and their management requires common sense. Because they are viral illnesses, they should not be treated with antibiotics. Flu symptoms are worse than cold symptoms and in some instances may lead to complications, but most healthy people recover from both colds and flu on their own with no need for drugs, prescription or OTC. Prevention is the best strategy. Those most at risk for complications from the flu should get the annual flu vaccine and should also ask a doctor about the need for prophylactic antiviral therapy. Wash your hands frequently, get plenty of rest and sleep, limit exposure to people who are already sick, and eat foods rich in antioxidant vitamins and minerals, such as brightly colored fruits and vegetables and dark, leafy greens. Add immune-boosting mushrooms, such as maitake and shiitake, to your favorite recipes, including chicken soup, which has been shown to help reduce the severity of cold symptoms. Consider taking additional vitamin C and vitamin D during cold and flu season, and perhaps trying astragalus or andrographis as well. If you do get sick, cough and sneeze into your sleeve and do not go to work or school until you are feeling significantly better, to reduce the chance of infecting others. Use gentle saltwater gargles to help relieve a sore throat; consider taking elderberry, Oscillococcinum, echinacea, or a pelargonium remedy; and ask your doctor about a prescription antiviral drug if the flu hits you particularly hard. Limit the use of OTC remedies and avoid combining multiple cold and cough products to lessen the risk of adverse events. If symptoms worsen or persist beyond ten to fourteen days, contact your doctor.

6

Sleep Aids

The best way to get an idea of how many of us are not sleeping well is to look at the extent of use of medications to treat the problem. It is estimated that 10 to 25 percent of Americans use prescription sleep aids, spending about $4.5 billion each year on them. Prescriptions for them jumped from 47 million in 2006 to 60 million in 2012 and have continued to increase since then. Women, the elderly, and highly educated people use more of them. And over-the-counter (OTC) products for sleep are some of the most popular items in pharmacies. I advise you to be wary of all these medications and knowledgeable about any you may be taking.

Here is one cautionary tale—with a happy ending.

Marjorie, a self-proclaimed type A personality, was a single parent and busy real estate agent when she first experienced occasional sleeplessness in her late thirties. She found herself gradually increasing her coffee consumption to make it through long days but then needed an extra glass of wine to slow down and get to sleep at night.

When she was in her forties, Marjorie experienced significant changes in her life: her only child left for college, she lost her beloved dog, and she began to have symptoms of perimenopause. She now felt "twired"— simultaneously tired and wired—throughout the day. And she struggled almost nightly with insomnia.

Marjorie's doctor believed that the insomnia resulted from a chemical imbalance common with aging and prescribed a low dose of zolpidem (Ambien), a popular sleeping pill. Her sleep improved at first, but Marjorie had to increase her dosage over time to maintain the drug's effectiveness. She felt groggy throughout her mornings and began discovering signs that she had been unconsciously eating in the middle of the night. When Marjorie tried to give up medication, her insomnia actually worsened; she was now dependent on zolpidem.

Marjorie turned to an integrative sleep medicine practitioner for help. He determined that a complex set of lifestyle, medical, and psychological factors were at the root of her insomnia and that the medication was only perpetuating the problem. Together, they devised a plan to simultaneously wean her from zolpidem and restore her natural sleep. The practitioner recommended a temporary course of natural sleep aids—valerian and melatonin—to support this transition.

Cognitive behavioral therapy (CBT) was a key component of treatment, with a focus on how Marjorie's thoughts, beliefs, and behaviors affected her sleep. It also addressed related lifestyle issues—her diet, exercise, and work and rest habits. She was advised to cut back her use of coffee during the day and wine at night and adhere to a regular sleep-wake schedule, with reduced light at night in her bedroom to make it more conducive to sleep.

Marjorie learned that like most people with insomnia she was *hyperaroused*—too stimulated by day to slow down and rest at night. She began a practice of mindfulness-based stress reduction (MBSR) to help manage this problem. She also began to see a counselor to deal with unresolved feelings of loss and loneliness, prompted by vivid dreams about her son and dog. Finally, after years of dreading the prospect of nightly struggles with insomnia, she started to sleep well again.

INSOMNIA

Insomnia refers to difficulty falling asleep, staying asleep, or obtaining restorative sleep. The National Sleep Foundation reports that 40 million Americans have a chronic sleep disorder and 62 percent of American adults experience a sleep problem a few nights a week.

Good sleep is a cornerstone of good mental and physical health. It restores energy and protects immunity. REM (rapid eye movement) sleep, the phase in which we dream, plays a critical role in learning, memory formation, and mood regulation. Poor sleep has been linked to chronic inflammation and increased risk for a broad range of illnesses, including depression, obesity, diabetes, cardiovascular disease, cancer, and autoimmune disorders.

The causes of insomnia are complex and intertwined with lifestyle. There are three types of factors—predisposing, precipitating, and perpetuating ones. Predisposing factors might include hyperarousal, the excessive use of substances like alcohol and caffeine, disruption of circadian rhythms (our twenty-four-hour cycle of physiological processes) through overexposure to light at night, and changes associated with aging. Precipitating factors refer to stressful events that push one over the threshold into insomnia. Examples include illness, divorce, menopause, and work or financial challenges. And perpetuating factors refer to misguided attempts at managing symptoms of insomnia, as by taking sleeping pills regularly. Medical conditions that cause pain or discomfort, or disrupt energy, as well as many commonly used medications, can also predispose us to, precipitate, or perpetuate insomnia.

Prescription Sleep Aids: How They Work, and Their Side Effects

Dozens of prescription drugs are marketed to treat insomnia. Benzodiazepines, a class of sedative anti-anxiety medications, are widely used at higher doses for insomnia. A number of other prescription sleep aids are known as Z-drugs, because the letter *z* appears in their generic names. Collectively, these medications are called sedative-hypnotics (from Hypnos, the Greek god of sleep). Although it's not their primary function, sedating antidepressants, antipsychotics, and antihistamines are also used "off label" as sleep aids.

Consumer cost of these drugs ranges from less than $1 to more than $30 per dose. The pharmaceutical industry promotes their sale through extensive direct-to-consumer ads and through contributions that influence public sleep education. For example, the National Sleep Foundation, the leading nonprofit organization dedicated to improving sleep health, has received substantial funds from numerous pharmaceutical companies.

Few people who rely on the most popular sleep aids understand how they work, their effectiveness (or lack of it), and their potential side effects and adverse reactions.

Although the use of herbs and alcohol to promote sleep dates back thousands of years, the first pharmaceutical sleep aids weren't developed until the nineteenth century. Barbiturates, a class of highly sedating and potentially dangerous drugs, came on the scene early in the twentieth century and dominated the sleeping pill market until the 1960s, when benzodiazepines (BDZs or "benzos") were introduced as a safer alternative.

BDZs are sedating medications that reduce anxiety, relax muscles, and promote sleep. The many drugs in this class differ in how rapidly they take effect and how long they continue working. Their generic names all end in "-pam" or "-lam," such as diazepam (Valium), alprazolam (Xanax), clonazepam (Klonopin), lorazepam (Ativan), triazolam (Halcion), and flurazepam (Dalmane). All work by boosting GABA (gamma-aminobutyric acid), a key neurotransmitter that calms brain activity. Since so much insomnia is associated with tension and anxiety, it's not surprising that BDZs help promote sleep. Whether taken for anxiety or insomnia, they can be miraculously effective when first used. Consequently, they are among the most commonly prescribed drugs worldwide.

BDZs are usually recommended for short-term use of two to four weeks, but many people take them regularly. Combining them with alcohol or other sedating drugs or with opioids is dangerous and potentially lethal. Common side effects of BDZs include drowsiness, loss of balance, dizziness, confusion, amnesia, and breathing difficulties. Although BDZs can help us fall asleep faster and stay asleep longer, they disrupt sleep architecture — our normal cycles of sleep and dreams. More specifically, they increase light sleep at the expense of deep sleep, and they suppress dream sleep (REM). Long-term use frequently results in tolerance — the need to increase the dose to maintain the desired effect — and dependence. Dependence on BDZs is particularly stubborn; some addiction experts say it is harder to overcome than addiction to opioids.

Z-drugs, the first medications specifically formulated to treat insomnia (approved in the 1990s), are also among the most popular sleep aids around the world. Prescriptions for Z-drugs rose 350 percent between 1999 and 2010. Like BDZs, Z-drugs increase GABA activity, but they are more selective in the brain areas they target. They are purported to have fewer side effects than BDZs and to not damage sleep architecture.

The major Z-drugs — zolpidem (Ambien), zaleplon (Sonata), and eszopiclone (Lunesta) — share a basic chemical structure, but they vary in terms of effectiveness, duration of activity, speed of onset, and side effects. Use of these Z-drugs has been linked to *parasomnias,* bizarre unconscious nighttime behaviors that include sleepwalking, sleep driving, sleep telephoning, sleep cooking and eating, and sleep sex. Other side effects are drowsiness, amnesia, headache, dizziness, and depression. Z-drugs should not be combined with alcohol or other sedating medications.

First developed in the 1950s, sedating antidepressants (SADs), including amitriptyline (Elavil), doxepin (Silenor), mirtazapine (Remeron), and trazodone (Desyrel), are extensively used to treat insomnia, although the US Food and Drug Administration (FDA) has not approved them for that. SADs are types of antihistamines, all of which cause drowsiness as a well-known side effect. Typically prescribed at low doses for insomnia, SADs are purported to be safe for long-term use. Although it's not entirely clear how it works, trazodone is one of the most popular sleep aids in use today and may be useful in treating insomnia caused by SSRI antidepressants (see chapter 9).

Sedating antidepressants have a potent anticholinergic effect, meaning they suppress the activity of acetylcholine, a key neurotransmitter. Many of their side effects are related to this activity: daytime sleepiness, weight gain, heart problems, digestive difficulties, headache, dry mouth, and blurred vision. SADs also aggravate restless leg syndrome and suppress REM sleep. These problems are of particular concern for the elderly, who generally use more anticholinergic drugs, such as allergy, antispasmodic, anti-nausea, and muscle relaxant medications. Overdosing on SADs is potentially lethal.

In addition to BDZs and SADs, other commonly used off-label sleep aids include antipsychotics, such as quetiapine (Seroquel) and olanzapine (Zyprexa); antiepileptics, such as gabapentin (Neurontin) and pregabalin (Lyrica); as well as an older antihistamine, hydroxyzine (Vistaril, Atarax). Although they share a common side effect of sedation, relatively little is known about their effectiveness and safety in the treatment of insomnia.

In recent years, ramelteon (Rozerem) and suvorexant (Belsomra), two new types of drugs that promote sleep in novel ways, have received FDA approval. Unlike other hypnotics, ramelteon promotes sleep by targeting brain receptors for melatonin, the neurotransmitter that regulates circadian rhythms. Designed to address sleep-onset difficulties, ramelteon is a relatively mild medication; nonetheless, side effects include daytime sleepiness, fatigue, concentration difficulties, headache, reduced libido, and fertility problems.

Suvorexant blocks the action of orexin (aka hypocretin), a neurotransmitter that promotes wakefulness. It was approved to treat insomnia in 2014 but not before the FDA considerably cut its proposed doses to reduce side effects. The most common of these are drowsiness, impaired driving, depression, suicidal thoughts, unusual dreams, hallucinations, and parasomnias similar to those seen with the Z-drugs. Suvorexant can also cause sleep paralysis, a frightening experience of being unable to move or speak for a few moments while falling asleep or awakening.

EFFECTIVENESS OF PRESCRIPTION SLEEP AIDS

Recent research using objective measures of sleep has raised serious questions about the overall effectiveness of sleep aids. On average, Z-drugs were found to reduce the time it takes to fall asleep by 13 minutes and add only 11 minutes to total sleep time. BDZs reduced sleep-onset time by 10 minutes and increased total sleep time by 32 minutes. And suvorexant decreased sleep-onset time by a mere 2.3 minutes, with an increase in total sleep time of 21 minutes. Although most of these improvements are statistically significant, they are functionally insignificant.

Also interesting is a discrepancy between these objective findings and subjective reports of satisfaction. Sleeping pill users estimated that their total sleep time increased by 52 minutes with BDZs and 32 minutes with Z-drugs. In all likelihood, the amnesia typically associated with these drugs interfered with remembering how badly they actually slept. Regular users of sleep aids also have more nighttime awakenings than insomniacs who do not use these products. When asked about this by a *New York Times* reporter, a representative of the pharmaceutical industry commented, "If you forget how long you lay in bed tossing and turning, in some ways that's just as good as sleeping."

OTC SLEEP AIDS

Each year, 10 to 20 percent of Americans take OTC sleep aids such as Zzzquil, Unisom, Nytol, Sominex, and various "PM drugs." Their popularity may stem from a belief that OTC products are safer than prescription sleep aids. Certainly, they are easier to obtain and cheaper. They are also capable of causing undesirable side effects.

Most OTC sleep aids contain antihistamines like diphenhydramine (Benadryl). Some also contain acetaminophen or aspirin. Like SADs, OTC sleep aids promote sleep by suppressing histamine. Common side effects include extended drowsiness, disorientation, constipation, urinary retention, blurred vision, dry mouth, and reduced REM sleep.

THE PROBLEMS WITH SLEEP AIDS

Apart from the many side effects and adverse reactions of sleep aids, there are other problems associated with their long-term use. For example, the residual "hangover" common with most of them can leave users impaired even when feeling fully awake. This can significantly increase the risk of motor vehicle accidents and falls, especially among the elderly.

Long-term use of BDZs, Z-drugs, OTC sleep aids, and especially SADs results in tolerance—the need to increase dosage to maintain the same effect. Tolerance encourages overmedication, in the form of both excessive dosing and the use of risky combinations of drugs and substances. History is replete with stories of celebrities who lost their lives to overmedication in a desperate pursuit of sleep. And, sadly, there are many more untold stories of ordinary people who did the same.

Although sleep aids purportedly treat insomnia, they are actually symptom suppressive—that is, they mask sleeplessness while failing to address its underlying causes. Consequently, discontinuation of these drugs often results in rebound insomnia, a recurrence and even worsening of one's original symptoms. Rebound insomnia can last from days to months, perpetuating dependence and addiction.

While the risk of tolerance, dependence, and rebound

insomnia is ostensibly lower with Z-drugs than with BDZs, in reality, the two are similar in terms of these adverse reactions. One significant disadvantage of BDZs is their potential for true addiction, with an extremely challenging withdrawal process. (See chapter 9 for the story of one woman's struggle with this.)

Never stop a sleep medication abruptly. It is much safer to taper the dose down gradually and under medical supervision. Depending on the type of drug, the dosage, and the length of use, sleep aid withdrawal can range from a minor bump in the road to a protracted ordeal lasting weeks or months. The withdrawal process is marked by symptoms that wax and wane, including rebound insomnia, anxiety, depression, and cognitive challenges.

While the long-term effects of Z-drugs on REM sleep are unclear, BDZs, SADs, and OTC sleep aids are known to suppress dreaming. These drugs have been linked to depression, dementia, and Alzheimer's disease, conditions also associated with impaired REM sleep.

More than a dozen studies have raised concerns about links between sleep aid use, cancer, and death rates. One study of more than ten thousand people who took Z-drugs or BDZs found a 35 percent increase in cancer rates as well as a correlation between increased use and death rates. Even people taking fewer than eighteen pills per year had increased mortality.

INTEGRATIVE MEDICINE APPROACHES TO MANAGING INSOMNIA

Despite widely publicized concerns about their safety and efficacy, sleep aids remain the most popular treatment for insomnia. This is reinforced by the medicalization of sleep — an industry-concocted notion that insomnia is caused by a chemical imbalance in the brain that can be remedied with a quick pharmaceutical fix. This perspective depersonalizes sleep. It discourages addressing critical personal and lifestyle issues and undermines our *sleep self-efficacy* — trust in our ability to heal our own sleep.

Like the common cold, occasional sleeplessness is transient and usually resolves on its own. But like a cold that persists, chronic insomnia should be treated professionally.

Because primary care practitioners generally do not have the training or the time to effectively address insomnia, they are more likely to prescribe sleep aids or refer patients for unnecessary overnight sleep studies. In contrast, behavioral sleep medicine (BSM) specialists are trained to address insomnia with personalized cognitive behavioral therapy for insomnia (CBT-I). A number of websites offer CBT-I programs that can be coupled with integrative medicine consultations.

Integrative medicine encourages a comprehensive

approach to insomnia rather than a purely chemical one. It relies on the principle of *endogenous healing*—a belief in our innate capacity and natural inclination to sleep. Instead of forcing people back to sleep with a drug, integrative medicine advocates the gentler approach of *invoking sleep*—with the active participation of the patient. Let's take a look at some of the methods used.

Noise Reduction

Most insomnia is not caused by insufficient sleepiness but by overstimulation arising from biomedical, psychological, and environmental factors or "body, mind, and bed noise." Noise reduction is about identifying and managing the kinds of excessive stimulation that interfere with our innate tendency to sleep.

Body noise refers to a wide range of biomedical problems that can contribute to sleeplessness. Examples include the adverse effects of caffeine or alcohol, pain or discomfort, digestive problems such as GERD, airborne and food allergies, symptoms of perimenopause, restless leg syndrome, and the side effects of medications. A lack of adequate physical activity as well as chronic muscle tension, which is usually rooted in anxiety, are also examples of body noise.

Conscientiously managing diet, substance use, and medical symptoms will help reduce body noise. It is also essential to evaluate the possible side effects on sleep of all medications you are using and consider alternatives as needed. Various mind-body techniques are available to help alleviate muscle tension: yoga, progressive muscular relaxation, breath work, self-hypnosis, transcranial stimulation, and neurofeedback. Mindfulness-based stress reduction (MBSR) is a structured form of meditation that has been shown to be very useful in improving sleep, as well as making it easier to taper off sleep aids.

Mind noise refers to sleep-impeding thoughts and feelings rooted in misguided beliefs. It is most effectively addressed with CBT-I, a set of techniques that help modify thoughts, beliefs, and behaviors that interfere with sleep. Although it does not work as quickly as sleep aids, CBT-I is significantly more effective and enduring. It commonly includes stimulus control and sleep restriction—two strategies that reduce insomnia by selectively limiting time in bed. CBT-I is particularly useful to mitigate excessive sleep effort, the common tendency of trying too hard to make sleep happen, which invariably backfires.

Integrative medicine also acknowledges the psycho-spiritual dimension of sleep. If there is a secret to falling asleep, it is the recognition that the awake part of us, by definition, simply cannot make it happen. In one sense, we never need to "go to sleep" because sleep already resides within each of us. We need, instead, to practice letting go of wakefulness. Mastering relaxation techniques, such as breath control, can help greatly.

Limiting use of computers, cell phones, and other forms of intrusive technology may be critically important.

Bed noise refers to such environmental factors as literal noise, excessive background light, poor air quality, and too-warm ambient temperature (above 68°F/20°C). A sleep-conducive bedroom should also feel safe—both physically and psychologically.

Herbal Remedies and Other Natural Products

Some botanical medicines and nutraceutical sleep supplements can help reduce insomnia as well as assist in withdrawal from sleep aids. In general, these products are both safer and less expensive than conventional sleep aids. They are best used as part of a comprehensive noise-reduction program. Although there is extensive information about natural sleep products on the Internet, I recommend seeking professional guidance—from a knowledgeable pharmacist or physician—about using them. Three of the most popular are valerian, L-theanine, and melatonin, all of which are well researched.

Valerian is a potent sedating herb that can support normal sleep architecture as well as deep and REM sleep. Used in many parts of the Western world for centuries, valerian has a good safety profile, but it should not be combined with other sedating substances or medications. It is best taken in the form of a standardized extract in capsules, 400 to 600 milligrams, a half hour before bedtime.

L-theanine is an amino acid with a good safety pro-file that effectively reduces anxiety and promotes relax-ation. Extracted from tea, it increases alpha EEG (relaxed brain waves) and increases GABA levels. Because anxi-ety is a common factor in sleeplessness, L-theanine can be helpful in treating insomnia. It can also counter some of the stimulating effects of caffeine. The usual dose is 200 to 250 milligrams.

Melatonin is a neurotransmitter that plays a key and complex role in our nighttime physiology by regulat-ing circadian rhythms and supporting healthy sleep and dreams. Available in a wide range of doses as well as regular and time-release formulations, it can help address various sleep concerns when used appropriately. Unfor-tunately, melatonin is often misunderstood and mis-used. Despite its good safety record, taking high doses will not necessarily help with, and might actually impede, sleep. Many dosage forms are available. I recommend 2.5 milligrams as a sublingual (under-the-tongue) tab-let at bedtime.

Bottom Line

Insomnia is a glaring symptom of an unhealthy life-style. Sleep aids suppress this symptom and replace it with counterfeit sleep that does not provide natural repose. Given their limited effectiveness, side effects, and serious adverse reactions, over-prescription and over-use of sleep aids are not justifiable. If they are to be taken at all, sleep aids are best used for short-term management of sleep problems, such as those related to emotional trauma (for example, a death in the family) or travel between different time zones. Safe and effective interventions that address insomnia as a lifestyle issue should always take precedence.

7

Steroids

Freddy Homburger, an oncologist as well as an enthusiastic watercolorist, admired the work of the acclaimed French painter Raoul Dufy long before he actually met the artist. It was, in fact, that admiration that brought the two men together. In 1949, Dr. Homburger saw a photograph in *Life* magazine of Dufy, then seventy-two years old, that showed the crippling effect of rheumatoid arthritis (RA) on the artist. Familiar with recent trials of adrenal hormone (cortisone acetate) in treating inflammatory conditions, he wrote to Dufy, explained the potential benefits and risks of participating in a clinical study of cortisone, and offered to admit him to his research unit in a Boston hospital should he decide to participate.

Having suffered from RA from his early youth, Dufy became increasingly disabled, could not stand without help, and struggled to paint, using only his left hand after losing the use of his right. (He had been unable to hold a brush for years; he had to attach it to his hand with tape.) Despite treatment with gold salts — the standard of the day — he continued to suffer severe flares that forced him to use crutches and finally a wheelchair. His work deteriorated markedly as a result of his illness.

Dufy accepted Homburger's offer and was admitted to Jewish Memorial Hospital in Boston in April 1950. After initial evaluation and treatment for gingivitis and poor dental health, he began receiving daily cortisone injections in dosages of 100 milligrams. Later, he was put on oral cortisone with buffered aspirin. To blunt the hormone's side effects, he was prescribed potassium supplements to counteract fluid retention and weekly testosterone to prevent osteoporosis, according to the medical standards of the time. (He was a heavy smoker and drinker, two habits that also promote bone loss.)

Despite fluid retention and stomach disturbances, Dr. Homburger noted that Dufy's response was "rapid, gratifying, and sustained." Records from the physiotherapy department showed that by mid-June, Dufy was able to resume many activities of daily living, which had been impossible on admission. Soon he could squeeze his paint tubes unassisted.

Dufy's joy in his progress was so great that his doctors suspected elevated mood due to the medication, but Berthe, his art dealer and lover, insisted that this was his "old self." She reported, too, that his libido had returned. With such improvement, a restless Dufy was released from the hospital to a hotel on the banks of the Charles River to paint. His daily cortisone dosage was reduced to 50 milligrams. Despite severe symptoms of toxicity—such as swelling of the face—he was now able to walk and paint for two to three hours a day.

In December 1950, Dufy developed an abscess in the left buttock at the site of his cortisone injections. Because of the ongoing hormone regimen, symptoms of infection were masked until the abscess became very large and Dufy began to show systemic signs: lassitude, malaise, and loss of appetite. Under anesthesia, more than 800 milliliters of pus were drained. Cortisone therapy continued.

On March 12, 1953, Dufy wrote in his last letter to Dr. Homburger, "I had an intestinal episode which appeared to take the form of an obstruction, today completely relieved. But I cannot help but feel a little disturbed about the future and will proceed henceforth with all precautions and remedies necessary."

Less than two weeks later, at the age of seventy-six, Raoul Dufy died from a massive intestinal hemorrhage, most likely a complication from his three years of continuous treatment with cortisone (and aspirin).

THE HISTORY OF STEROIDS

The story of cortisone is synonymous with Dr. Philip Showalter Hench, of the Mayo Clinic in Rochester, Minnesota. In April 1949, Hench shared startling images of patients with RA; all had recovered with synthetic cortisone. His discovery was hailed as a genuine miracle cure. The following year, Hench and his associate, Edward Kendall, received a Nobel Prize for "discoveries relating to the hormones of the adrenal cortex, their structures and biological effects."

As the most powerful anti-inflammatory agent yet discovered, cortisone transformed the practice of rheumatology almost overnight. It also revolutionized ophthalmology, gastroenterology, respiratory medicine, dermatology, and nephrology (kidney disorders), and facilitated two remarkable postwar therapeutic developments: organ transplantation and treatment of childhood cancers.

Cortisone and its derivatives, now collectively known as *steroids* (or *corticosteroids*), remain among the top ten most widely used prescription and over-the-counter (OTC) drugs. They remain the most powerful anti-inflammatory agents known, and their significance in general medicine is beyond dispute. The number of patients treated with them and their range of clinical applications exceed those of all other medications. It is not surprising that steroids are included in the World Health Organization's Model List of Essential Medicines.

Millions of new prescriptions for oral steroids are written each year in the United States alone. An estimated 1.2 percent of the US population over the age of twenty—more than 2.5 million people—received oral steroids between 1999 and 2008. While significant, these numbers fall short of total corticosteroid use, as many more people are taking these drugs by topical application and inhalation.

Given practically any disease of unknown cause for which there is no effective treatment, physicians will often put patients on a trial of cortisone to see what happens. The simple convenience of writing a prescription for a steroid has supplanted the traditional scientific method of first understanding a disease and then developing an effective treatment for it.

STEROID DRUGS

Hormones produced by the adrenal cortex (the outer layer of the adrenal gland) consist of four carbon rings linked to form what chemists call the *steroid nucleus.* Variations on this molecular theme result in drugs with greater or lesser anti-inflammatory potency and more or less of the undesirable effects of salt and water retention.

In 1955, prednisone was introduced into clinical medicine as the first synthetic steroid drug, and three years later, triamcinolone was patented. Prednisone is about five times stronger than cortisone but has the same salt- and water-retaining properties. Triamcinolone is as powerful as prednisone but has less propensity for salt and water retention. When triamcinolone is dissolved in acetone, the resultant triamcinolone acetonide (Trianex, Triesence, Triderm) is very potent and, as a fat-soluble compound, is easily absorbed through the skin, making it the preferred topical steroid in creams and lotions for dermatitis and psoriasis. Intramuscular injection of triamcinolone is sometimes used to control allergic asthma, severe contact dermatitis, seasonal allergic rhinitis (hay fever), and transfusion and drug hypersensitivity reactions (serum sickness). In 2014, the US Food and Drug Administration (FDA) allowed over-the-counter sale of triamcinolone acetonide in nasal spray form under the brand name Nasacort.

Triamcinolone joint injections (Kenalog) for osteoarthritis and RA offer rapid pain relief, usually within twenty-four to forty-eight hours. Improvement lasts six to twelve weeks on average, and injections can be done safely two to three times a year. (In my experience, their efficacy lessens over time.)

HOW STEROIDS WORK: A DOUBLE-EDGED SWORD

Although inflammation can be troublesome, it is actually the cornerstone of our healing system — the body's way of getting more nourishment and more immune activity to an area that is injured or under attack by germs or toxins. The body regulates inflammation carefully: too little creates susceptibility to infection; too much causes tissue damage and increases risks of allergy and autoimmunity. The twin adrenal glands and the hypothalamus and pituitary in the brain produce very potent hormones that regulate the inflammatory response as well as general metabolism, bone and muscle health, and heart, liver, and kidney function. These hormones also strongly influence our mental and emotional life.

Steroids, either produced in the body or taken as medication, bind tightly to glucocorticoid receptors present in virtually all cells in the human body. This interaction then regulates gene expression in the cell nucleus, suppressing inappropriate inflammation in many tissues and organs: for example, in joints, where inflammation causes RA; in nerves, where it leads to neurological disorders; or in the airways, where it causes asthma. The most important effects of steroids result from these *genomic* mechanisms. They occur at all dosages, even very small ones (low-dose therapy), and they happen relatively slowly—it may take up to eighteen hours for steroids to take genomic effect.

But at higher doses, *non-genomic* effects come into play rapidly—over seconds or minutes—resulting from direct interactions with biological membranes. These interactions influence nerve function in the brain, affecting hormone production, behavior, and cognition. This is an important distinction, because the relative potencies of various steroids are completely different in terms of producing non-genomic versus genomic effects.

Uses of Steroids

Steroids can be lifesaving in cases of allergic (anaphylactic) shock and other severe allergic reactions, in the treatment of autoimmune diseases, in cases of brain swelling, in cancers of the blood and lymphatic system, and in transplant medicine to prevent rejection of donor organs. In these instances, their worth as immunosuppressant and anti-inflammatory agents is undisputed. But steroids are now used for a great many other conditions, some of them far from serious—like minor cases of dermatitis from contact with poison oak and ivy, diaper rash, and ordinary aches and pains. It is not a good idea to use such powerful drugs for routine complaints. Most people who use steroids do not understand how they work and how dangerous they can be.

When initiating steroid treatment, experts agree on using the smallest dose for the shortest time. Criteria for effectiveness and ineffectiveness of treatment must be defined at the outset, so that treatment can be stopped if it is not helping. Typical doses of prednisone (or its equivalent) are as follows:

- Low dose: less than 7.5 milligrams per day
- Medium dose: 7.5 milligrams to 30 milligrams per day
- High dose: more than 30 milligrams per day

Bear in mind that even small doses of steroids (less than 5 milligrams daily) may cause problems.

The Problems with Steroids

Dose, duration, route of administration, and form of the steroid all influence the frequency and severity of adverse events, as do the patient's condition and medical history. In 1950, at the age of seventy-three, Raoul Dufy was the oldest patient ever to be treated with cortisone. His age, smoking, drinking, and daily aspirin use all increased his susceptibility to steroid toxicity. He suffered from salt and water retention, facial swelling (often referred to as "moon face," occurring as a result of redistribution of body fat), infection, mood disturbance, and chronic stomach irritation that led to a fatal gastrointestinal bleed.

Common adverse effects of oral steroids include the following:

acne
blurred vision
cataracts or glaucoma
depression
difficulty sleeping
high blood pressure
increased appetite and weight gain
increased growth of body hair
lowered resistance to infection
muscle weakness
nervousness and restlessness
osteoporosis
sudden mood swings
swollen, puffy face
thinning of skin and easy bruising
worsening of diabetes

Adverse effects are less frequent with steroid injections but can include these:

allergic reactions
bleeding into the joint
infection at the site of injection
skin discoloration
weakening of bone, ligaments, and tendons (from
    frequent, repeated injections into the same area)

Between 1997 and 2014, the FDA received reports of ninety serious neurologic events, some fatal, related to epidural injection of steroids — a procedure commonly performed to manage neck and back pain. In 2014, the FDA issued a class warning that "safety and effectiveness of epidural administration of corticosteroids have not been established."

Inhaled steroids, widely used for management of asthma, have fewer adverse effects than oral steroids, but they can cause hoarseness and promote fungal infection of the mouth and throat (thrush). Rarely, prolonged use of inhaled steroids in high dosage will cause the same systemic toxicity seen with long-term oral steroid therapy.

Topical steroids can have local or, rarely, systemic side effects. The stronger the medication, the larger the area to which it is applied, and the longer it is used, the more likely that adverse effects will occur. Young children and the elderly are more susceptible, because they tend to have thinner skin. Topical steroids can cause these side effects:

acne or worsening of existing acne

burning, stinging, or irritation of the skin

changes in skin color

excessive hair growth

inflamed hair follicles

rosacea

stretch marks

thinning of the skin

worsening of a preexisting skin infection

One other concern: because steroids suppress symptoms of disease rather than treating root causes, long-term use may strengthen disease patterns and encourage their spread to other sites. For example, suppression of allergic dermatitis in children with long-term topical steroid treatment may increase the risk of later development of asthma. Autoimmune diseases typically wax and wane and have a high potential to go into remission. Long-term immune suppression with steroids may decrease the likelihood of remission. In other words, steroids provoke powerful homeostatic reactions, natural processes aimed at maintaining consistent conditions internally. This pattern can lead to tolerance — the need for larger doses over time — and stubborn dependence that encourages persistent use. Long-term use of steroid drugs is always associated with adverse effects, many of them quite serious.

Perhaps, the most noteworthy fact about steroids is

that they are *pleiotropic,* meaning that they have multiple effects on diverse biological functions. Doctors prescribe them and people take them to alleviate symptoms caused by excessive or misdirected inflammation, but they also suppress immunity in general, increasing susceptibility to infection and retarding wound healing. Over time they regularly cause adverse effects in many systems, from irritation of the stomach to loss of bone density and disturbances of mood.

Sudden discontinuance of steroid therapy or too-rapid lowering of dose usually results in immediate return of symptoms, often worse than before the start of therapy. Because of the homeostatic rebound problem, one should never stop steroid treatment abruptly or decrease the dose too quickly. The weaning process must be slow, and should start only after other measures are in place, such as dietary change and use of natural anti-inflammatory agents. Of course, nonsteroidal anti-inflammatory drugs (like aspirin and ibuprofen) are available as alternative medications, but these have their own drawbacks with long-term use (see chapter 8).

Oral prednisone tablets, 5 to 60 milligrams per day, cost less than $25, with similar figures for oral methylprednisolone (Solu-Medrol) and triamcinolone. Despite the low price of oral steroids, costs associated with adverse effects can be a significant component of the total cost of treatment with these drugs.

INTEGRATIVE MEDICINE APPROACHES TO MANAGING INFLAMMATORY DISORDERS

Integrative medicine offers a number of strategies for managing unwanted inflammation and misdirected immunity, beginning with dietary change.

The body synthesizes substances that regulate inflammation from essential fatty acids (those we cannot make and must get from dietary sources). In general, the omega-6 fatty acids that are found in seeds, grains, nuts, and vegetable oils are the precursors of substances that increase inflammation, while the omega-3 fatty acids, found mostly in oily fish, are the precursors of substances that tamp it down. We need both kinds of fatty acids in the right proportions to keep the inflammatory process in balance. Too little inflammation leaves us susceptible to infection; too much pushes us toward allergy, autoimmunity, and all the diseases associated with excessive, purposeless inflammation. The mainstream diet is top heavy in omega-6s from the refined vegetable oils used in processed foods, and deficient in omega-3s. Correcting this imbalance—by decreasing intake of processed foods and increasing intake of cold-water oily fish and supplemental fish oil—can make a big difference in inflammatory status.

The mainstream diet promotes inflammation in other ways, too: it gives us quick-digesting forms of carbohydrates and not enough of the protective elements found in fruits, vegetables, herbs, and spices. Integrative medicine practitioners routinely recommend an anti-inflammatory diet to many patients on steroids. This type of diet avoids processed foods, limits sugar and animal protein (except for fish and high-quality dairy products), makes liberal use of extra-virgin olive oil, and includes fruit in moderation and an abundance of vegetables. Often, these dietary changes are enough to enable patients to begin weaning themselves off steroids.

Nature provides several powerful anti-inflammatory agents that are nontoxic, not suppressive, and safe for long-term use. Chief among them is turmeric *(Curcuma longa)*, the spice that gives its deep yellow color to curry powder and prepared yellow mustard. An impressive body of scientific evidence documents its anti-inflammatory properties. A botanical relative, ginger *(Zingiber officinale)* is also effective, and the two can be used together. Although both fresh and powdered turmeric and ginger can be added to foods, for medical use, standardized extracts are better. The reishi mushroom *(Ganoderma lucidum)*, used for centuries in traditional Chinese and Japanese medicine, is another effective, natural anti-inflammatory agent. Too woody and bitter to eat, it is best used in the form of extracts, either liquids or capsules. Follow the dosage recommendations on these products.

The brain and nervous system influence immune

function and inflammation. This is the subject of a robust field of study known as *psychoneuroimmunology*. Reducing stress, practicing relaxation techniques, and employing mind-body therapies (hypnosis, guided imagery, mindfulness training) can dramatically impact inflammatory diseases.

Additional nonpharmacological interventions are available to manage symptoms for which steroids are commonly used. Acupuncture and osteopathic manipulative therapy (OMT), for example, can relieve many kinds of musculoskeletal pain. Traditional Chinese medicine is often able to change the course of ulcerative colitis, Crohn's disease, and other autoimmune conditions. There are safe and effective botanical remedies for common allergies (see chapter 4), as well as simple home remedies for contact dermatitis and other skin problems. (One example: running hot water for a few minutes—as hot as one can tolerate—on the rash of poison oak or ivy will cause the itching to intensify immediately, then subside for a long time; doing this whenever itching begins hastens resolution of the outbreak.)

BOTTOM LINE

Steroids have been the focus of high hopes and heated debate ever since their dramatic effect on rheumatoid arthritis was discovered more than half a century ago. Certainly, they have a secure place in the medical practice of the present and future. But just as certainly, they are widely overused, often for trivial conditions, and often as the sole or principal treatment for problems that could be managed more safely and as effectively by other means. They are routinely used long term, causing dependence and significant toxicity. Save these powerful drugs for serious medical conditions and try to slowly wean off them once improvement occurs by instituting other measures to keep symptoms at bay.

8

Nonsteroidal Anti-Inflammatory Drugs (NSAIDs)

I would be surprised if you do not keep a supply of aspirin in your home and probably also ibuprofen. These and other nonsteroidal anti-inflammatory drugs (NSAIDs) are among the most widely consumed medications today. They can be miraculously effective at relieving pain, lowering fever, and reducing swelling associated with inflammation. Over-the-counter (OTC) forms are so familiar that most people consider them totally benign and take them frequently or even regularly with little awareness of their risks.

Salicylic acid, the precursor of aspirin, is a constituent of willow bark, a folk remedy used for centuries in diverse parts of the world. Hippocrates prescribed willow bark tea for headache 2,400 years ago. Aspirin was synthesized in 1897. Today, it is one of the most widely used medications in the world, with an estimated 40,000 tons of it consumed each year. In the 1960s, the first non-aspirin NSAID was introduced: indomethacin (Indocin), a prescription medication still used today. Currently, there are at least twenty prescription-only formulations, as well as a multitude of brand-name and generic versions of OTC NSAIDs; aspirin, ibuprofen (Advil, Motrin), and naproxen (Aleve) are familiar examples.

But these widely used drugs are not benign, as the following story of a patient illustrates.

Angela, a sixty-six-year-old woman, made a New Year's resolution to lose some extra pounds and get in better shape. Her weight had increased over the past ten years due to a more sedentary lifestyle after she was diagnosed with osteoarthritis of her knees and lower back. She had been taking anti-inflammatories (600 to 800 milligrams of ibuprofen) to control her pain. In the past month, Angela started to attend Zumba (dance fitness) classes twice a week. Initially, her aches and pains worsened, so she doubled her dose of ibuprofen most days. For the past week, Angela has experienced unusual fatigue and trouble catching her breath when she climbs the stairs in her house. Today, she pushed herself to go to her Zumba class and developed chest pain when she started moving. Her instructor called 911, and she was brought by ambulance to the emergency room, where she was found to be profoundly anemic from bleeding gastric ulcers, requiring admission to the hospital, cardiac monitoring, and transfusion.

Angela's serious adverse gastrointestinal effect from taking an OTC anti-inflammatory medication is—unfortunately—not uncommon. Through her hospital experience, she realized she needed to find alternative methods to address her pain, including dietary change and other lifestyle modifications, as well as more gentle physical activity before going back to high-impact exercise. She found a health provider to help her select appropriate integrative treatments to decrease pain and improve her general well-being.

How Nonsteroidal Anti-Inflammatories Work

Like Angela, a great many adults in the United States take anti-inflammatory medications prescribed by health professionals or purchased over the counter. The class of medications called NSAIDs includes a large number of pain- and fever-reducing drugs. Notable anti-inflammatory medications *not* in this class are prednisone and acetaminophen (Tylenol). Prednisone is a steroid (see chapter 7); acetaminophen is an OTC drug that reduces pain and fever by a different mechanism than that of NSAIDs. NSAIDs come in many forms:

long-acting, short-acting, injectable; in liquids and tablets; and as creams, gels, and patches for topical application. They are often included in cold and flu remedies.

NSAIDs fall into two categories, selective and nonselective, based on how they work. All NSAIDs act at the level of cells by inhibiting an enzyme called COX (cyclooxygenase). There are two forms of the enzyme: COX-1 is produced constantly in the tissues, whereas COX-2 is elicited mainly by inflammation. Both are involved in making prostaglandins, regulatory compounds found in every tissue that modulate our response to injury. It is prostaglandins that directly cause pain, fever, and more inflammation. Blocking their synthesis decreases those responses. Most NSAIDs, including aspirin and ibuprofen, are non-selective in that they block both forms of the COX enzyme. Unfortunately, their suppression of COX-1 also increases the risk of gastrointestinal ulceration and bleeding, the main adverse effects of these medications. Selective COX-2 inhibitors were developed to reduce those problems. Celecoxib (Celebrex), a prescription NSAID, is now the only selective NSAID still available. Two other selective NSAIDs were removed from the market in 2004 and 2005 due to increased risk of heart attack and stroke.

Topical NSAIDs have some effect on pain and inflammation, though less than oral forms. When applied to the skin, some of the drug is absorbed into the tissue at the site of application. Patches and gels can cause local irritation, but because little of the drug is absorbed into the bloodstream, overall they are a less risky option, with far fewer adverse effects than oral forms. OTC Aspercreme contains a milder relative of aspirin, trolamine salicylate, which has a minimal effect on pain; some preparations combine it with lidocaine, a topical anesthetic.

The cost of NSAIDs varies widely—from $4 a month for a generic OTC product to $1,500 a month for a brand-name prescription drug. There are few differences among the non-selective NSAIDs, whether OTC or by prescription. Except for Aspercreme, topical NSAIDs are still available only by prescription and range in price from $196 to $498 per tube.

Common Uses of NSAIDs

Common conditions treated with anti-inflammatory medications include back and neck pain, joint pain associated with various types of arthritis (such as rheumatoid arthritis, osteoarthritis, gout, and psoriatic arthritis), chronic muscle and body aches and pains, musculoskeletal injuries (fractures, tears, or strains), menstrual cramps, headaches, and fever, among others. Daily low-dose aspirin is used to aid in the prevention of stroke, heart attack, and some forms of cancer (esophageal and colorectal, for example) — most appropriately in people with preexisting disease or significant risk factors. The risks and benefits of a low-dose aspirin regimen for prevention should be discussed with a health professional; they vary, depending on age, bleeding risk, current medications, and other health conditions.

NSAIDs can be particularly problematic when used daily for chronic pain because of the side effects described above. In low to moderate doses for short periods of time (days to weeks), they can greatly reduce pain and inflammation without significant risk, as long as blood pressure is well controlled, and there is no kidney disease, heart disease, intestinal ulceration, or known gastrointestinal inflammation. When used daily for more than a few weeks, the likelihood of serious adverse effects increases.

Inflammation is the body's normal response to injury and leads to swelling, pain, and sometimes heat and redness. This response is beneficial: it lets us know that we have been injured and that we need to protect the affected body part. Furthermore, the inflammatory response promotes healing by bringing more blood, nutrients, and immune activity to an injured site. NSAIDs can decrease the inflammatory response after trauma to bones, joints, muscles, or tendons, rapidly reducing pain and swelling. When left untreated, serious injuries can develop into chronic pain syndromes due to compensations by other body parts to protect the injured part and to changes in the brain. Other types of inflammation and pain syndromes that occur in the body can result from daily "wear and tear," inactivity or over-activity, stress, and chronic illness. Because NSAIDs do not treat the root causes of chronic pain syndromes but simply suppress symptoms, they may, over time, intensify or prolong the problem by allowing people to continue the activities that have caused it. (See chapter 12 for more information on medications for chronic pain.)

Recent research has shown chronic inflammation to be associated with depression, and trials of NSAID therapy as a novel treatment for severe depression suggest that it works better than antidepressant drugs in some patients.

THE PROBLEMS WITH NSAIDs

Despite being highly effective at reducing acute and chronic pain, fever, and inflammation, all NSAIDs come with significant risks. The side effects and adverse reactions caused by them impact the stomach, intestines, heart, lungs, blood vessels, and blood cells. Individuals vary in susceptibility to these, based on their health status and disease risks.

The most significant and common adverse effects of NSAIDs occur in the gastrointestinal (GI) tract. Many users will experience stomach pain, flatulence, or some type of stomach irritation with only one dose. The real potential for harm comes with daily use, generally for more than two weeks. When NSAIDs get into the bloodstream and block the COX-1 enzyme, synthesis of prostaglandins decreases. Among other functions, these hormone-like substances protect the stomach lining from acid and other irritants. Over time, deficiency of prostaglandins increases the possibility of gastric bleeding, ulceration, and perforation, any of which can occur in the absence of warning symptoms. Thousands of people die each year from episodes of NSAID-related GI bleeding; many of them had no awareness of the harm the drugs were causing. The decrease in prostaglandins can also damage the small and large intestines, especially in the setting of ulcerative colitis and Crohn's disease. (The selective COX-2 medication celecoxib has a lesser impact on the GI tract, though it is not entirely without risk.)

NSAIDs also affect our blood cells, particularly platelets. Platelets protect the walls of blood vessels by binding to them to patch holes and keep blood from leaking out of arteries and veins. Aspirin acts in a unique way: it blocks platelets from clumping together to form clots for the entire life of the platelet, which is eight to twelve days. Ibuprofen and other NSAIDs exert this effect for a much shorter time. In the case of a heart attack, platelet blocking is desirable; in other instances—such as an upcoming surgery, intestinal bleeding, or a low platelet count to begin with—it is potentially dangerous.

All these risks need to be considered when deciding whether or not to take aspirin or other NSAIDs.

Aspirin is routinely given to patients who are having a heart attack, and low daily doses of it have been shown to help prevent both heart attacks and strokes. Regular use of NSAIDs other than aspirin can increase blood pressure, worsen heart failure, and increase the risk of death from heart disease. Much research has looked at this. Naproxen (Aleve) appears to increase heart attack risk least and diclofenac (Voltaren) most. The COX-2 inhibitor celecoxib, despite having lower gastrointestinal risk, is the worst of all NSAIDs when it comes to heart disease. Anyone at high risk for heart disease and stroke should avoid it.

NSAIDs also impact the kidneys, which need prostaglandins produced by the COX-2 enzyme to maintain the blood flow that keeps them healthy and functioning. Because all the NSAIDs block this enzyme and decrease renal blood flow, those with kidney disease should not take them. Even in the absence of kidney disease, those who take diuretics ("water pills") for heart failure or hypertension should be careful, because the combined effects of diuretics and NSAIDs can cause kidney problems.

Drug Interactions

The major category of drugs that can interact with NSAIDs is blood thinners. When taken with any blood thinner, especially warfarin (Coumadin), NSAIDs will increase the risk of GI bleeding. Alcohol intake on its own increases this risk; together with regular use of NSAIDs, alcohol multiplies it. Long-term use of corticosteroids, such as prednisone, can cause stomach ulcers; combined with NSAIDs, the risk is amplified.

The pharmaceutical antidepressants known as selective serotonin reuptake inhibitors (SSRIs), such as fluoxetine (Prozac), sertraline (Zoloft), and paroxetine (Paxil), decrease platelet clumping in a different way from NSAIDs. When NSAIDs and SSRIs are taken together, the risk of bleeding increases. Herbal remedies and supplements that affect platelets and should be avoided by those on NSAIDs include danshen *(Salvia miltiorrhiza),* dong quai *(Angelica sinensis),* evening primrose oil, and willow bark.

INTEGRATIVE MEDICINE APPROACHES TO TREATING ACUTE INJURY, CHRONIC INFLAMMATION, AND PAIN

Rest, ice, compression, and elevation of an acutely injured limb or body part as soon as possible will decrease swelling and pain and speed recovery. Topical application of tincture of arnica *(Arnica montana),* as long as the skin is not broken, is also helpful and can reduce bruising.

Lifestyle Change

Lifestyle change is the most useful approach when trying to manage chronic pain syndromes associated with inflammation. Improved diet and exercise can lead to weight loss, and weight loss often reduces chronic pain by decreasing the workload on joints, especially in the knees, hips, and back. In women with hormone-related migraine, exercise helps by lowering estrogen levels.

The single most effective strategy is adopting an anti-inflammatory diet. Over the course of weeks to months, it can decrease inflammation, promote weight loss, and alleviate chronic pain. The anti-inflammatory diet focuses on a diversity of fresh vegetables and fruits, whole grains (as opposed to products made with flour), healthy fats (extra-virgin olive oil in particular, which contains a unique anti-inflammatory compound called oleocanthal), seeds and nuts, oily fish, whole soy foods, healthy herbs and spices (especially turmeric and ginger), tea (white, green, or oolong), and occasional healthy sweets such as dark chocolate or dried fruits. Many of these foods have been shown to decrease chronic inflammatory markers in the body. Notably missing from the anti-inflammatory diet pyramid are many of the foods commonly consumed in the standard American diet (referred to as the SAD diet in some health circles), especially processed and manufactured foods, which are major sources of pro-inflammatory fats and carbohydrates (sugar and flour). Except for fish, eggs, and high-quality dairy products, animal foods are minimized.

Exercise is one of the best-studied treatments for pain. This can include physical therapy following injury (after the swelling has reduced and a professional has cleared the patient for exercise), as well as routine exercise and stretching programs to improve function. Activities like yoga, Pilates, and tai chi can help large-joint pain; walking or swimming can improve sciatic pain and lower back pain; and weight training can strengthen muscles that surround problematic joints, decreasing pain by reducing the burden on the joints themselves. It is important to start exercise slowly and build up steadily. Exercise is also one of the best treatments for insomnia, and it is well established that improved sleep can result in decreased chronic pain.

Smoking is associated with increased chronic pain, including lower back pain, and quitting smoking is likely to result in improvement.

Nutritional Supplements and Botanicals

Several herbal remedies and dietary supplements have been shown to decrease inflammation and treat pain. Arnica can be applied topically, as mentioned above, to the site of an injury to reduce pain and swelling. It has also been shown to decrease pain and swelling after surgery. Additionally, arnica has been shown to decrease pain associated with mild to moderate osteoarthritis. Capsaicin cream is another useful topical product that can decrease pain, particularly nerve pain, as from peripheral neuropathy or an outbreak of shingles. Capsaicin is the compound that gives hot peppers their heat; it can initially cause a mild to moderate burning sensation. The greatest effects are felt after several weeks of use.

Fish oil supplements have consistently been found to decrease chronic inflammation and pain, including arthritis pain, neuropathy, and menstrual cramping. Turmeric is the most powerful natural anti-inflammatory; both the whole spice and its main active component—curcumin—have been shown to decrease inflammatory markers and improve chronic pain associated with inflammation. In fact, curcumin supplementation has been found to be as effective as ibuprofen for osteoarthritis of the knee, without any of the troubling side effects of that drug. Extracts of a familiar relative of turmeric—ginger—have been shown to modestly improve pain associated with osteoarthritis of the knee.

Other Therapies

Manual therapies such as massage, chiropractic, and osteopathic manipulation can be effective for chronic pain management. Most research using these modalities has focused on lower back pain. Acupuncture can also work as an alternative to chronic NSAID use for a number of painful conditions, including menstrual cramps, chronic lower back pain, joint pain, dental pain, and migraine or tension headache.

Mind-body approaches, such as hypnosis, guided imagery, and guided meditation, can provide relief by teaching patients to change their perception of painful sensations.

Clearly, there are a number of possibilities to help manage pain before reaching for an anti-inflammatory medication.

BOTTOM LINE

Widespread use and easy availability of nonsteroidal anti-inflammatory drugs promote the mistaken belief that these drugs are perfectly safe. Many people take them regularly and thoughtlessly. In fact, they are powerful medications with significant potential for harm when used long term. For chronic pain syndromes, they should never be the sole treatment. Integrative medicine offers many ways to manage chronic pain, so that NSAIDs are required intermittently or not at all.

9

Psychiatric Medications for Adults

Olga is a seventy-year-old woman with resistant depression. She had been hospitalized several times for severe depression and anxiety. During the most recent hospitalization, after forty sessions of electroconvulsive therapy (ECT), she had been sent home with prescriptions for multiple medications. These included quetiapine (Seroquel), an antipsychotic drug used to stabilize mood and control anxiety; lamotrigine (Lamictal), an anticonvulsant used mainly for bipolar disorder; and clonazepam (Klonopin), an anti-anxiety agent. Olga had been on many other psychotropic medications in the past. None of them really helped, and all gave her intolerable side effects: dry mouth, nausea, headache, increased anxiety and depression, insomnia, decreased sex drive, and fatigue. On the current medication regimen she felt very tired and sedated but no less depressed and anxious. Her psychiatrist suggested that she receive another course of ECT, which Olga wanted to avoid due to its negative effects on her memory. Refusing this treatment, Olga found her way to an integrative psychiatry clinic.

After a comprehensive evaluation of her history, an examination of her mental status, and a discussion of her options, Olga received a course of acupuncture treatment twice a week, along with weekly psychotherapy. The latter combined cognitive behavioral therapy (CBT) and Neuro-Emotional Technique (NET), a mind-body therapy based on Chinese medical philosophy. Acupuncture reduced the anxiety and depression. Cognitive behavioral therapy helped Olga become aware of her distorted thinking and develop better coping skills, while the NET lessened her habitual reactions to past traumatic life experiences.

After three months, Olga was free from most of her depressive symptoms. She was able to reduce her dosages of Seroquel and Klonopin and discontinue the Lamictal completely. Supplemental nutrients, including omega-3 fatty acids and vitamin D, were prescribed to improve brain function, which further helped relieve her depression and anxiety. Olga's emotional health is not yet optimal; she still needs a low dose of Seroquel at night and occasional Klonopin to help buffer the overwhelming stress in her life. But she is no longer depressed and is much more socially active. It is expected that in the next six to twelve months, Olga will continue to improve and possibly discontinue all medication.

The Biomedical Model in Psychiatric Medicine

The word *psychiatry* derives from Greek roots meaning "soul doctoring"—a noble enterprise. Sadly, psychiatry today has lost touch with its roots. It is now dominated by the biomedical model, which attributes all disturbances of mental and emotional health to imbalances of brain biochemistry, correctable by medication. Big Pharma has taken great advantage of this by marketing an array of drugs to treat depression, anxiety, and major mental illnesses. Looking at the ads for these products in medical journals, one would think that these conditions would no longer exist, that by taking the medications everyone would be enjoying optimum emotional health. In practice, however, the drugs discussed in this chapter fall short of the promises made for them by their manufacturers—often dramatically so.

Psychotropic drugs are capable of affecting the mind, emotions, and behavior. The main classes of psychotropic medications are antidepressants, atypical antipsychotics, and anti-anxiety agents. They are widely used to treat depression, anxiety disorders, and other conditions marked by abnormalities of thought, mood, and behavior, sometimes for just a few months but more often for long-term, even lifelong, treatment, despite their potential for harm. Psychotropic medications account for 48 percent of the severe adverse drug reactions that affect millions of people in the United States. (Adverse reactions to drugs are the fourth leading cause of death in our country.) Nevertheless, global sales of psychotropic drugs have reached more than $76 billion a year.

ANTIDEPRESSANTS

The Centers for Disease Control and Prevention (CDC) reports that about 9 percent of adult Americans suffer from depression. And 3 percent of adults have major depressive disorder, a long-lasting and severe form that is the leading cause of disability for Americans between the ages of fifteen and forty-four.

Antidepressants supposedly improve the symptoms of depression by impacting the brain chemicals (neurotransmitters) associated with emotion — serotonin, norepinephrine, and dopamine. Newer medications with better side-effect profiles — selective serotonin reuptake inhibitors (SSRIs) and serotonin norepinephrine reuptake inhibitors (SNRIs) — have replaced the older tricyclics and monoamine oxidase inhibitors (MAOIs).

Some SSRIs and SNRIs are also used for anxiety disorders, mostly fluoxetine (Prozac), sertraline (Zoloft), citalopram (Celexa), duloxetine (Cymbalta), and venlafaxine (Effexor). Doctors prescribe them to avoid long-term use of benzodiazepines, the anti-anxiety drugs that too often cause stubborn dependence and addiction. Doctors also prescribe these medications "off label" to treat chronic pain, menstrual symptoms, low energy, migraine, irritable bowel syndrome, and other conditions.

The CDC reported that from 2005 to 2008, 11 percent of Americans were taking a prescription antidepressant. In 2010, antidepressants were the second most commonly prescribed medications, just behind cholesterol-lowering agents, costing us almost $10 billion.

The rate of antidepressant use across all age groups exploded from 1988 to 2008, increasing nearly 400 percent. One study showed that medical professionals other than psychiatrists wrote 80 percent of antidepressant prescriptions, often without a specific psychiatric diagnosis.

Aggressive direct-to-consumer marketing of these drugs certainly accounts for much of their popularity. Big Pharma has convinced many people that ordinary states of sadness represent imbalances in brain chemistry that antidepressant medications can correct. But a growing body of data suggests that for mild to moderate depression, the drugs are no more effective than placebos.

THE PROBLEMS WITH ANTIDEPRESSANTS

Long-term use (more than a year) may prolong or intensify depression, a phenomenon called *tardive dysphoria*. That's medical jargon for "lingering bad mood," resulting from the body's homeostatic reaction to the medication: if you keep a patient on a drug that increases serotonin at neural junctions, over time the brain will compensate by producing less serotonin and fewer serotonin receptors, making things worse.

Questionable efficacy aside, antidepressants commonly cause sexual difficulties, interfere with concentration, and disturb digestion. Less frequent side effects include increased risk of relapse, liver toxicity, decreases in bone mineral density, abnormal bleeding, stroke, and suicidal behavior. Several studies have shown that especially in older people, antidepressants are associated with an increased risk of death from all causes. Use by pregnant women may increase the risk of autism in their children, as well as birth defects.

ATYPICAL ANTIPSYCHOTICS

Antipsychotics are intended to treat schizophrenia and related serious mental illnesses. They work mainly by regulating the neurotransmitter dopamine. The newer, so-called second-generation antipsychotics (SGAs), also known as atypical antipsychotics, have been marketed since 2000. Examples of atypical antipsychotics are aripiprazole (Abilify), clozapine (Clozaril), ziprasidone (Geodon), olanzapine (Zyprexa), quetiapine (Seroquel), and risperidone (Risperdal). Although they have a better side-effect profile, the efficacy of SGAs is not as good as that of the first-generation drugs, such as chlorpromazine (Thorazine) and haloperidol (Haldol).

While the incidence of illnesses for which antipsychotics are indicated has not increased, the use of these drugs has skyrocketed. In 2011 alone, they were prescribed to 3.1 million Americans at a cost of $18.2 billion, a 13 percent increase over the previous year. The number of annual prescriptions for atypical antipsychotics rose from 28 million in 2001 to 54 million in 2011, a 93 percent increase. In 2013, Abilify was the number one prescribed psychotropic medication and the overall top drug by sales, bringing $6.5 billion to the company manufacturing it. Between 2001 and 2011, the US Veterans Health Administration and

Department of Defense spent almost $850 million on Seroquel.

The dramatic increase in the use of these drugs dates from 2003, when the FDA approved their use as adjunctive therapy for severe depression. Direct-to-consumer advertising campaigns by the drug companies increased from $1.3 billion in 2007 to $2.4 billion in 2010; more than 98 percent of all advertising of atypical antipsychotics was spent on just two drugs: Abilify and Seroquel, the current best sellers. They are now commonly given along with SSRI antidepressants as first-line treatment, probably with the hope that they will improve the often less-than-stellar benefits of those drugs. Furthermore, physicians prescribe these medications off label for insomnia, anxiety, stress, and mild mood disorders, all of which makes me uneasy.

THE PROBLEMS WITH ATYPICAL ANTIPSYCHOTICS

The SGAs can cause severe adverse reactions, including sudden cardiac death and blood clots, as well as increased risk of stroke and diabetes. More importantly, long-term use of antipsychotic medication does not provide more benefits than short-term use and may actually hinder patients' return to a healthy work and family life.

Anti-Anxiety Medications

Anxiety disorders affect about 18 percent of the adult population, or 40 million people eighteen years or older in the United States in any given year. They include obsessive-compulsive disorder (OCD), post-traumatic stress disorder (PTSD), generalized anxiety disorder (GAD), and phobias. Together, they cost the United States more than $42 billion a year, almost one-third of the country's $148 billion total mental health bill.

A variety of medications are prescribed to treat the symptoms of anxiety disorders. Benzodiazepines, such as alprazolam (Xanax), lorazepam (Ativan), and diazepam (Valium) are used for generalized anxiety disorder and panic disorder. Heart medications known as beta blockers reduce the physical trembling and sweating that people with phobias experience in difficult situations. Antidepressants, both old and new, are now approved for treating OCD.

Benzodiazepines ("benzos") appear to work by enhancing the effects of the calming neurotransmitter GABA (gamma-aminobutyric acid) in the brain. Because they work quickly and can be very effective in the short term, benzos are widely used to treat anxiety, seizures, insomnia, muscle tension, alcohol withdrawal and drug-associated agitation, nausea, and vomiting. A 2013 survey showed that Xanax has consistently been the number one prescribed psychiatric medication, with Ativan at number five and Valium in eleventh place.

THE PROBLEMS WITH ANTI-ANXIETY MEDICATIONS

Anti-anxiety medications have many serious and common side effects: unusual sleep behaviors, cognitive deficits (including loss of ability to form new memories), impairment of driving and other daily activities, and increased risk of falling, particularly in the elderly. Severe allergic reactions to them have also been reported. Other side effects can include low blood pressure, decreased sex drive, nausea, lack of coordination, disinhibition, depression, anger, and violent behavior. Moreover, it is easy to become dependent on benzos. Many people who take them regularly find they have to increase the dose to maintain the desired effect and cannot stop taking them because of severe rebound of their symptoms. Benzo dependence is harder to break than opioid addiction; withdrawal can be life threatening. Discontinuation of a benzodiazepine must be done gradually and only under a doctor's direction.

I consider these drugs some of the most overused and misused pharmaceutical products, and I find it appalling that doctors prescribe them casually and for long-term use with little regard to their potentially devastating effects on memory and other cognitive functions and their addictive potential. I feel so strongly about this that I want to relate the story of a patient I worked with recently as she struggled to free herself from dependence on Ativan.

Rachel first experienced panic attacks at the age of fifty. They were infrequent, and she did not know the cause. A physician friend and colleague recommended that she take a low dose of Ativan (0.5 milligram) to manage the attacks. She did not take it often but gradually found that she liked the feeling she got from it and thus began to take it even in the absence of a panic attack. At age fifty-eight, Rachel was working hard in a high-stress job. She felt anxious most of the time, had disturbed sleep, and suffered migraines twice a week.

When she turned sixty, Rachel left her job. Then her marriage fell apart, leading to what she described as a "total physical and mental breakdown," with increasing anxiety. She started taking the low dose of Ativan every night, but still her anxiety worsened. The same physician advised her to take an additional 0.5 milligram dose once or twice a day, followed by the bedtime dose. Following a divorce and a move, she was put on an antidepressant (Zoloft) that she stayed on for two years.

After five years of taking no more than 2 milligrams of Ativan a day, Rachel's anxiety continued to increase, especially first thing in the morning. She recalls that her "whole life became about managing anxiety." At this time she was also smoking a lot of marijuana, taking Tylenol with codeine recreationally, and drinking alcohol nightly. She worried about cognitive impairment from the Ativan, because her "mind was not working right" and decided she should get off it. She sought help from a psychiatrist, but he did not see discontinuing the Ativan as a priority. Instead, over the ten months that she was in treatment with him, he insisted on focusing on her relationship with her mother rather than on her drug use. Another physician friend also made light of Rachel's concerns about Ativan, and her brother, a neurosurgeon, told her, "Ativan can't be causing your problems; millions of people take it."

But another friend, a psychologist, suspected she might be having rebound anxiety in the morning—a withdrawal reaction as the previous night's dose wore off. The possibility that the Ativan might now be causing and intensifying her anxiety made sense to her and solidified her motivation to stop taking it. At that point she came to me for help. I taught her a calming breathing technique and recommended that she take kava (Piper methysticum), a safe and effective herbal relaxant and anti-anxiety agent. I also sent her to a sleep therapist and had her talk to a colleague who specializes in addiction treatment. On her own, Rachel stopped using marijuana and Tylenol with codeine and reduced her intake of alcohol. She then began a detox program, using a liquid form of Ativan that she could dispense by drops in order to gradually decrease the amount she was taking. She took kava twice a day for anxiety and did a lot of acupuncture for insomnia.

One day, about two months into the program, Rachel reported, "I suddenly felt clear—as if a screen lifted between me and reality." Shortly afterward, her anxiety began to dissipate. It took her four months to get off the Ativan completely. The constant anxiety that had plagued her for so long never returned. She says, "It is astonishing to me that my dependence on Ativan actually prolonged and intensified my anxiety and that until I saw you, none of the doctors I consulted warned me of the dangers of using it regularly."

OPTIMAL USE OF PSYCHOTROPIC MEDICATIONS

Psychotropic medications may help reduce depression and acute anxiety, especially when counseling and other measures are employed, but they don't work for everyone.

It is better to start with only one medication at a time, beginning with a low dose, to minimize the risk of side effects and interactions. The longer someone is on a psychotropic medication, the harder it is to stop it, as the patient's brain chemistry becomes adapted to the drug over time. It is not advisable to stop any psycho-tropic medication abruptly—better to taper off slowly while instituting other measures.

Except in the case of bipolar disorder and other major mental illness, it is unwise to rely on psychotropic med-ications long term without addressing the complex causes of the conditions being treated.

INTEGRATIVE MEDICINE APPROACHES TO MANAGING MOOD DISORDERS

The complexity of mental illnesses and their underlying causes requires an individualized, integrative approach, rather than an effort to simply try to correct a presumed imbalance in brain chemistry through treatment with drugs.

Psychopharmaceutical therapy based on the bio-medical model assumes that a molecular abnormality in the brain is the cause of a clinical syndrome; there-fore, correcting such an abnormality with medication is the solution. However, multiple genetic and environ-mental factors participate in the development and sustainment of mental illness. When these factors are addressed, patients may experience better outcomes and suffer fewer side effects. They may be able to cut the number of drugs they are taking and reduce dos-ages, eventually discontinuing all psychotropic medication. This approach must be individualized and well coordinated by an integrative psychiatrist to make sure it is done safely and effectively.

Many options are available for managing depression and anxiety without drugs. There is good scientific evidence, for example, for the antidepressant effects of exercise and supplemental fish oil (to provide the essential omega-3 fatty acids needed for optimal brain function). Talk therapy, especially CBT, often works as well as or better than medication to treat depression. Acupuncture can be useful as well. Learning to regulate the breath is a more effective anti-anxiety measure than benzodiazepines, without any of the cognitive impairment and addictive potential of those drugs.

An integrative assessment for mental and emotional problems should look at dietary habits; use of alcohol, caffeine, and other psychoactive substances; physical activity; sleep patterns; and issues with work, social relations, and more. Treatment recommendations might include lifestyle modifications, dietary supplements, herbal remedies and other natural products, and psychotherapy.

BOTTOM LINE

The drugs discussed in this chapter should not be used as first-line interventions for the most common mental/

emotional health problems. Antidepressant drugs are indicated for major depression, not for routine management of mild to moderate depression, for which more effective and safer treatment options exist. Even in cases of severe depression, use should be limited to a year at most. If you are taking antidepressant medication, never stop it suddenly; if you want to get off it, taper the dose slowly and only after instituting other measures to stabilize mood.

Try to avoid anti-anxiety drugs except for short-term management of situational anxiety, such as that associated with a death in the family, job loss, or other emotional upheaval. If you have been on a benzodiazepine for more than a month, consult a knowledgeable physician about discontinuing it.

10

Psychiatric Medications for Children and Adolescents

School kids lining up in class to get their meds like patients in a psych ward? Yes, it's now an everyday event, and most of the pills being dispensed are prescription psychiatric medications: psychostimulants for attention deficit hyperactivity disorder (ADHD), anti-anxiety agents, antidepressants, and even antipsychotics, to make the antidepressants work better. What have we come to?

Here is the story of one family's experience with these drugs.

"I want the old Marisa back," cried her mother, as she sat with her thirteen-year-old daughter and told the pediatrician her story. Over the past four months, Marisa had been making superficial cuts on her wrists with a razor blade. She was isolating herself, sleeping and eating poorly, and having thoughts of not wanting to live, as well as skipping school to avoid the embarrassment of experiencing her daily panic attacks in class. Her mom had looked for a therapist but learned it would be a two-month wait, and then insurance would cover only eight sessions. The wait to see a pediatric psychiatrist was even longer. The pediatrician started Marisa on a widely used antidepressant—escitalopram (Lexapro), a selective serotonin reuptake inhibitor (SSRI). After a few days on the drug, Marisa felt "revved up" and antsy and had even more difficulty falling asleep. A few weeks later, at their next appointment, the doctor reassured mother and daughter that these were temporary side effects and recommended adding quetiapine (Seroquel), an antipsychotic medication often used in low doses to help with sleep and anxiety.

There was progress. The Seroquel helped Marisa sleep and reduced her anxiety so that she was able to resume school after having missed two full weeks. But she now had a hard time waking up in the morning and felt exhausted all day. Her appetite increased, too. These are all common side effects of Seroquel. A few weeks later, Marisa reported that while she didn't feel as depressed as she had felt before, she also didn't "really feel anything anymore." Along with the other side effects, this emotional "numbness" bothered her so much that she stopped both medications abruptly. A few days later,

Marisa experienced common SSRI withdrawal symptoms: nausea, headache, flu-like aches, and lightheadedness. And her difficulty sleeping returned.

It turned out there were deeper issues that the drugs never touched. Months later, when Marisa's mom finally got her in to see a therapist, Marisa was able to describe the distress of growing up with parents who fought constantly. Her father struggled with anger and alcohol abuse. Eventually, her parents separated, but a few months before she had received an unexpected Facebook message from her dad telling her he would be moving back to their town. This news reawakened frightening memories that kept Marisa awake at night. On top of feeling exhausted from lack of sleep, she felt sick to her stomach and uninterested in food. Fortunately, therapy helped. Marisa joined a Mind-Body Skills Group for teens at a local community center, where she learned to use mindfulness, music, movement, and breathing techniques to calm herself and get to sleep; she also tried imagery, journaling, and art to work through her unresolved fear, grief, and anger. All these non-pharmacological approaches helped her regain emotional health.

Mental health issues are prevalent today, among children and teenagers as well as adults. The Centers for Disease Control and Prevention (CDC) reports that approximately one in five children in the United States experiences a mental disorder in any given year. Conditions include ADHD; autism; anxiety, depressive, bipolar, and psychotic disorders; obsessive-compulsive disorder (OCD); and eating and substance abuse disorders. The costs add up to more than $240 billion in annual spending to cover health care, educational services, and decreased productivity. Diagnoses are made using specific criteria when the child's ability to learn, behave, handle emotions, or function is significantly impacted. The causes of these disorders are not completely clear; both genetic and environmental factors are thought to contribute.

The use of psychiatric medications for children and adolescents is rapidly increasing in the United States and internationally. According to the US National Health and Nutrition Examination Survey, 6 percent of US teens reported using a psychiatric medication in the past month: 3.2 percent were prescribed antidepressants; 3.2 percent, medications for ADHD; and 1 percent, antipsychotics. Additionally, mood stabilizers (lithium, valproic acid [Depakote], and others) are often used for aggression and bipolar disorder, although there is limited information on the effectiveness or safety of this group of medications in children and teens. A 2014 report from the Agency for Healthcare Research and Quality (part of the US Department of Health and Human Services) showed that out of the $117.6 billion spent on medical care for children in 2011, the largest expenditure was for the treatment of mental health disorders—$13.8 billion, with 41.5 percent going toward prescription medication.

Medications rarely cure childhood mental illness; at best, they manage emotional and behavioral symptoms. When symptoms are severe, medications may be an important part of a comprehensive treatment plan, with the risk of side effects deemed acceptable for the short-term benefits. Too often, however, there is a lack of adequate and appropriate resources in the child's life and in the mental health system to address the contributory environmental components and behavioral patterns. As in Marisa's case, finding a helpful therapist may take months, and insurance coverage may be inadequate. Psychiatric medications seem like a quick and easy fix—the intervention that doctors turn to first and the one that parents have been led to believe is best.

At present, psychiatry is ruled by the biomedical model, which attributes all disturbed mental and emotional function to imbalances in brain chemistry, treatable with drugs. If this were the whole story, psychiatric drugs would be much more effective than they are. Pharmaceutical companies exaggerate their benefits and downplay their risks in marketing them to both doctors and the public.

The focus of this chapter is antidepressant, antipsychotic, and anti-anxiety medications as they are used in children and adolescents. For a discussion of drugs for ADHD, see chapter 11.

Antidepressants

Nearly 20 percent of adolescents will have experienced depression by age eighteen. If unaddressed, depression can increase the risk for legal difficulties, drug abuse, physical illness, and problems with school, work, and social functioning. Of greatest concern is the increased risk for suicide, the second most common cause of death among fifteen- to twenty-four-year-olds.

Prior to the 1990s, the only medications available to treat depression had not been shown to be effective in children and were not recommended for them because of significant safety concerns. When the first SSRI, fluoxetine (Prozac), came on the market, it was found to be effective for the treatment of depression in seven- to seventeen-year-olds. SSRIs increase the chemical serotonin in the spaces between brain cells. Many SSRIs are now widely prescribed: sertraline (Zoloft), paroxetine (Paxil), citalopram (Celexa), and escitalopram (Lexapro). SSRI use by children and teens has increased dramatically in the past two decades. A related category of medications, serotonin norepinephrine reuptake inhibitors (SNRIs), affects both the neurotransmitters serotonin and norepinephrine. Examples of SNRIs are venlafaxine (Effexor), desvenlafaxine (Pristiq), and duloxetine (Cymbalta), among others.

But how effective are these drugs in children and teens? A group of studies pooled together showed that, overall, 61 percent of the children and adolescents receiving antidepressants improved (defined as a 50 percent reduction in symptoms), compared to 50 percent of those given a sugar pill. (That is fairly good efficacy for the sugar pill, by the way, and it causes no adverse reactions.) In depressed children twelve or younger, antidepressants were found to be less effective than in adolescents. For treating anxiety disorders they tend to be more effective: the group receiving medication registered approximately a 70 percent improvement, as opposed to 40 percent in the placebo group.

The Problems with Antidepressant Use in Children

Like Marisa, 20 to 45 percent of youth experience side effects within a few weeks of starting an antidepressant: restlessness, irritability, agitation, insomnia, aggression, and mood swings. Fortunately, these resolve when the medication is discontinued. Side effects from SSRIs can involve more than behavior, though. For example, preliminary research associates use of them with decreased bone mineral density. Given that adolescence is a crucial time for bone development, this effect could have lifelong consequences.

As in Marisa's case, many children and teens stop taking their drugs because of their unpleasant side effects. Some of these are well known; others are not as well documented. For example, both SSRIs and SNRIs alter chemicals that play key roles in brain development. Most studies of their effects on the developing brain have been conducted in animals. For example, lab rats were given Prozac in adolescence, then observed as adults after discontinuing the Prozac. Compared with placebo treatment, the rats given Prozac before maturity show less despair when faced with stress, but they also react with more anxiety. Also, these rats show problems with sexual behavior as adults, even after the drug has long since been discontinued. Many adult humans experience sexual side effects from antidepressants; however, little research has been done in this area with children and teens.

What about prescribing multiple psychiatric medications to children? For example, many children are diagnosed with both depression and ADHD and then are treated with an SSRI antidepressant and a psychostimulant such as methylphenidate (Ritalin). No research exists on the long-term safety of this drug combination in children, but animal research suggests that it might be detrimental, especially in high doses. We know nothing about the long-term effects of combining medications early in life for humans; the concern is that medication exposure during childhood may have far-reaching consequences in adulthood.

Before the 1960s, bipolar disorder was hardly recognized in children, but by the 1990s, its incidence had exploded, much more than in adults. Was this sudden increase due to a real increase in prevalence, to better reporting, to applying the diagnosis more broadly, or perhaps to an ill-advised trend toward giving psychiatric medications to young people? We don't know. A study of children diagnosed with bipolar disorder found that about 60 percent had been treated previously with an antidepressant or a stimulant medication. It is unclear if these children would have developed the disorder anyway or if the medication precipitated an illness that otherwise would not have surfaced.

In 2004, the US Food and Drug Administration (FDA) issued a "black box" warning against the use of antidepressants in children and teens. This action was based on data suggesting a twofold increase (4 percent for those receiving antidepressants compared with 2 percent on placebo) in suicidal thoughts and behaviors when antidepressants were prescribed to youth who were not previously suicidal. Although the increased risk may be small, given the seriousness of suicide, this finding calls for judicious use of antidepressants, and close monitoring.

Marisa described feeling "numb" a few weeks after she started an SSRI, a common reaction. Some people may find the reduced intensity of both pleasant and unpleasant emotions helpful, but for others, it may feel quite limiting—by making them unable to cry when feeling sad, for example, or to experience joy. The cause and prevalence of this side effect, especially in young people, are not known, but this is another concern, since it is in childhood and adolescence that we learn to process emotions.

ANTIPSYCHOTICS

Over the past two decades, the use of antipsychotics to treat children's and teens' emotional and behavioral symptoms has skyrocketed. In 2010 alone, approximately one million US children and adolescents were prescribed antipsychotic drugs. Originally indicated for major mental illnesses, they are now commonly given along with SSRIs as first-line interventions for depression in adults, probably to compensate for the often less-than-stellar efficacy of SSRIs. While these medications can reduce symptoms of psychosis, mania, aggression, insomnia, and anxiety, they have significant side effects. Antipsychotics fall into two main groups: first-generation antipsychotics (FGAs) and second-generation antipsychotics (SGAs). SGAs are the main category prescribed to children and teens.

They affect dopamine and serotonin processing and include medications such as risperidone (Risperdal), olanzapine (Zyprexa), quetiapine (Seroquel), ziprasidone (Geodon), aripiprazole (Abilify), iloperidone (Fanapt), paliperidone (Invega), lurasidone (Latuda), asenapine (Saphris), and clozapine (Clozaril).

In the United States the various SGAs are FDA-approved for use in children and teens with schizophrenia, bipolar disorder, and irritability associated with autism. However, the majority of SGAs are prescribed off label for depression, anxiety, insomnia, and disruptive behavior — without much being known about their long-term risks versus benefits. Only a small percentage of children and teens who are prescribed these powerful drugs also receive psychotherapy.

THE PROBLEMS WITH ANTIPSYCHOTIC USE IN CHILDREN

SGA side effects are more common in children than in adults, affecting many systems. Nervous-system side effects include drowsiness, seizures, and abnormal movements. Some studies even suggest a reduction in brain volume over time from the use of these medications. The endocrine system can also be affected, with changes in levels of hormones that influence growth and development, sleep, mood, metabolism, and sexual function. Marisa's appetite increased once she began taking Seroquel; most SGAs cause significant weight gain within a short time. For example, in one study, Abilify use resulted in a weight gain of 10 pounds after eleven weeks; Zyprexa, 19 pounds; Seroquel, 13 pounds; and Risperdal, 12 pounds. SGAs also raise the risk of type 2 diabetes, and they increase blood levels of cholesterol and the hormone prolactin, with the latter being especially problematic after puberty. High prolactin is associated with amenorrhea (cessation of menstruation), galactorrhea (milk production in the breasts in the absence of pregnancy and childbirth), reduced sexual desire, erectile dysfunction, and osteoporosis.

Again, the long-term safety of these medications is not the only concern. Because SGAs can reduce emotional symptoms, they are often used without any attention paid to the complexity of factors that contribute to mental health problems in children, such as poor nutrition and sleep, unresolved or ongoing trauma, lack of consistent parenting, underdeveloped social- or emotion-regulation skills, and mismatches between teaching style and a child's learning needs. A growing number of experts feel that the risks of antipsychotic medications in children and teens outweigh the benefits and that much of their current use is inappropriate.

ANTI-ANXIETY AGENTS: BENZODIAZEPINES

Benzodiazepines are best known for producing calming, sleep-inducing, anti-anxiety, anti-seizure, and muscle-relaxant effects rapidly—within minutes to hours. Popular drugs in this class include alprazolam (Xanax), diazepam (Valium), clonazepam (Klonopin), and lorazepam (Ativan). Benzodiazepines have not been approved by the FDA for use in children and adolescents with mental health concerns. The few trials conducted to evaluate them as treatment for pediatric anxiety (school refusal, generalized anxiety, and separation anxiety disorder) have been small and of poor quality and have shown no more benefit than placebos. Nonetheless, they are sometimes prescribed, off label, based on benefits seen in adults.

THE PROBLEMS WITH BENZODIAZEPINE USE IN CHILDREN AND ADOLESCENTS

Side effects include a "dulling" effect on the mind, reduced short-term memory, increased agitation in some children, dependence, and withdrawal symptoms (insomnia, irritability, increased anxiety) when the dose is lowered or stopped.

Given that teens are one of the highest-risk groups

for abusing pharmaceuticals, the addictive potential of benzodiazepines should be of great concern. Adolescence is a time of novelty seeking. Without proper tools to cope with distressing emotions and situations, teens are likely to look for ways to numb their anger, fear, or grief. Once they experience the "Xanax feeling," they are more likely to seek it out repeatedly. In one study, teens prescribed benzodiazepines were ten times more likely to misuse these medications to get high (compared to teens never prescribed) and three times more likely to use someone else's prescription.

LIMITATIONS OF PSYCHIATRIC MEDICATIONS IN CHILDREN AND ADOLESCENTS

The causes of emotional and behavioral problems in young people are complex. From the time of conception, genetic and environmental factors play critical roles in the development of the child's nervous system. Pregnancy and birthing stressors, exposure to drugs and toxins, parental mental illness and family discord, childhood nutrition, sleep, and physical activity all play a part in how well a child can cope with life stress without falling ill. Adequate playtime and creative outlets, a sense of love and belonging, as well as structure and healthy boundaries all contribute to the mental health of children. In contrast, traumatic experiences in early life (emotional, physical, or sexual) can adversely impact mental health for years to come. Teasing apart all these contributing factors takes time and considerable patience, often not allowed for in the current medical model. No drug or combination of drugs can "make it all better."

From conception on, the brain goes through significant growth and change. Brain cell connections are initially overproduced. Later, during adolescence, these extra connections are "trimmed" back to help the brain adapt to the needs of the environment, a remodeling process that stays fluid until about age twenty-five. We have no idea how psychiatric medications affect brain development and what might be the long-term consequences of their use in early life.

INTEGRATIVE MEDICINE APPROACHES TO MANAGING MOOD DISORDERS IN CHILDREN AND ADOLESCENTS

To fully address the mental health issues of children and teens, an integrative approach is necessary. Every child must deal with an important ongoing challenge: how to manage emotional and behavioral responses when faced with higher demands and responsibilities. It requires learning and practicing healthy ways to express and move through emotions without getting stuck in them. Stress itself is not unhealthy; however, stress in excess of support can cause distress and illness. When challenge is balanced with supportive resources, children can attain an increasing sense of mastery that allows them to thrive. Emotional and behavioral symptoms in children are not necessarily problems to be eradicated; it may be more useful to view them as red flags, warning of issues needing attention.

Nutrition is among the most important yet easily overlooked factors in the mental health of children. A diet of unprocessed whole foods, with a predominance of fresh vegetables and fruits, plant-based protein, and fish, with minimal to no sugar, white flour, preservatives, and artificial colors, limits inflammation in the body and promotes better mental health. (Recent research links depression with increased inflammation.) Transitioning a child with mental health struggles to such a diet is an important step in treatment. Supplementing with omega-3 fatty acids (fish oil) and vitamin D can further support brain function.

Adequate restful sleep is another essential. A healthy bedtime routine might include soothing music, a warm bath, use of calming essential oils (especially lavender) and herbal teas (such as chamomile), a meditation practice, guided imagery, and appropriate reading. Optimal sleep requires reduction of excessive lighting, noise, and screen-related activities (TV, video games, cell phone) for two hours prior to bedtime. Removal of caffeine is important, as it disrupts the sleep cycle and can cause or worsen anxiety.

Another crucial element is regular physical activity, proven to enhance mood and sleep. Exercise need not be limited to participation in organized sports; indeed, joyful movement can consist of various forms of dance, yoga, jumping on a trampoline, or walking the dog. Engaging in play, spending time in nature, and enjoying quality time with friends and family are all essential. Children and teens require healthy daily routines, encouragement, and discipline. Without a sense of stability and structure, kids are much more likely to stay stuck in unhealthy emotional and behavioral patterns.

Therapies such as cognitive behavioral therapy (CBT), which can help a child or adolescent recognize and change unhelpful negative thought patterns, and techniques such as deep breathing to relax the mind and body can be as useful as antidepressant medications for some children. Because such approaches build skills for expressing and regulating emotions and improve awareness of thought and emotion patterns, they tend to have more lasting effect than medications used alone.

Family therapy can help children and their families become aware of unhealthy communication or coping patterns and learn to practice better ways of relating. Therapy groups that teach children and teens about fun and functional ways to regulate their emotions (using art, music, movement, journaling, and personal and group reflection, for example) can help build skills for controlling emotions and improving social interactions. In safe small-group settings, kids can more easily learn how to express and process difficult feelings.

BOTTOM LINE

Children and teens are not little versions of adults—their brains and bodies are not fully developed. For this reason, medications that work for adults are not necessarily effective or safe in kids. We do not have the research to know the long-term effects of the drugs, their influence on the developing brain, or the safety of combining them. To put it bluntly, we are doing a vast experiment with our children in maintaining so many of them on psychiatric medications.

In the context of an integrative treatment plan, medications can be a catalyst for positive change when addressing mental health issues. The risks of untreated symptoms must be weighed against the side effects of drugs and their potential for long-term harm. When medication is used, side effects can be minimized by beginning with a low dosage and increasing it slowly; this will also allow time to gauge efficacy. Medication treatment should always be integrated with psychotherapy and other non-pharmacological approaches and should be discontinued as soon as possible, although it is important not to stop the drugs abruptly as this can cause unpleasant withdrawal reactions.

Investment in the well-being of children is key to the future of our world. Although our current system and approaches help the mental health of many children and teens, staggering numbers remain symptomatic. It is unreasonable and dangerous to think that psychiatric medications can solve this problem.

11

Medications for Attention Deficit Hyperactivity Disorder (ADHD)

Attention deficit hyperactivity disorder (ADHD) is another condition that did not exist when I was growing up. It is now epidemic in North America, and we are successfully exporting it, or at least the idea of it, to other parts of the world. To the extent that it is a legitimate diagnosis — in my opinion it often is not — the causes are complex. It may result from a mismatch between individuals' styles of learning and working and the environments in which they are expected to learn or work. Dietary and other lifestyle factors may be involved. But, consistent with the tendency to medicalize behavioral and emotional problems, ADHD is now thought to be rooted in an imbalance of brain chemistry best treated with medication.

Nine-year-old Maya was having trouble in school. She was mildly hyperactive and had difficulty focusing on assignments, especially reading and writing. She also had a hard time sitting without fidgeting and often annoyed the teacher by talking to classmates and blurting out answers impulsively. In spite of this, standardized testing showed her to be in line with her peers at the fourth-grade level academically.

At home, Maya was a sweet and loving child who had some difficulty staying focused on routine tasks. Homework was often a battle, as she tended to avoid starting it and became distracted easily. Yet she loved both drawing and painting and could concentrate on them for hours. She was also an avid and skilled soccer player, although her distractibility sometimes greatly irritated her coach. She was popular and had good friends.

Her school history was inconsistent. Teachers had noticed her difficulties as early as kindergarten, with some years much harder than others. Her second-grade teacher had urged Maya's parents to have her evaluated for ADHD and start medication. They consulted their pediatrician, who spoke with them for fifteen minutes and asked them and the teacher to fill out questionnaires. When these were returned, the pediatrician stated that Maya had ADHD and suggested a "trial" of Concerta, a long-acting form of methylphenidate (Ritalin). Her parents were reluctant and decided to wait.

In third grade, although Maya's behaviors were similar, her teacher did not seem bothered and was able to get much more work out of her with positive reinforcement and a few simple accommodations. But her fourth-grade teacher told the parents that she was "not fulfilling her potential" and insisted on treatment. So Maya started taking Concerta. For the first few months, things seemed much improved. She was able to focus better both at home and at school, and the teacher was happy with her progress. The drug decreased her appetite and she lost a little weight. She was also more irritable, especially after school, when she would fly off the handle easily in a way that she never had before. A few times she complained of seeing odd things that were not visible to her parents. They felt, however, that the improvements in school outweighed these negatives.

Then, a few months later, Maya's former third-grade teacher contacted the parents and said that when she observed Maya around the school, the child seemed "a little flat." Could she be depressed? The parents were upset at this and, after watching more carefully, felt that she indeed might be depressed. They decided to stop the Concerta, which, they felt, was responsible. Within days, Maya returned to being the happy and joyous girl they remembered. Her mother's exact words were, "It was as if the Concerta had been a dam that was holding back her happiness." Maya did not restart the drug, and her parents found other ways to manage her ADHD.

THE CONTROVERSY

Attention deficit hyperactivity disorder is easily the most controversial condition in pediatric medicine.

It is defined as a neurodevelopmental disorder characterized by hyperactivity, difficulties with focus or attention, and impulsivity. Although many people have some of these traits, the symptoms must be severe enough to impact two separate areas of life to justify the diagnosis. For children this is usually home and school. From being an uncommon syndrome affecting less than 3 percent of the population in the 1970s, the prevalence of ADHD has risen dramatically. Currently, about 11 percent of children — about 6 million — in the United States have been diagnosed with it. And according to the latest government statistics, about 4.2 million of them are taking a psychostimulant medication like Ritalin for the problem. ADHD is the most common chronic disease of childhood, even more prevalent than asthma. Recently there has also been a dramatic rise in the diagnosis of ADHD in adults.

There is great controversy, both inside and outside

the medical profession, about whether the dramatic rise in prevalence represents a true increase in the number of people who have this syndrome or whether it is an epidemic of overdiagnosis. More extreme skeptics question the very existence of ADHD. Once given the diagnosis, the majority of children will be treated long-term with psychostimulant medication, in line with the recommendations of the American Academy of Pediatrics and other medical authorities.

I believe ADHD to be a real condition, with significant consequences for those most severely affected, but I also believe that it is greatly overdiagnosed, thanks to many factors, but especially to the high demands on and lack of support for our children. It defies common sense that 11 to 15 percent of all children (fully 20 percent of our boys) have suddenly become afflicted with a condition requiring lifelong medication.

A thorough discussion of how this has happened would fill the pages of an entire book. Here are just a few issues that illustrate the inaccuracy and capricious nature of our diagnostic approach.

In 2010, a researcher showed that children born in August were more than twice as likely to be diagnosed with ADHD and treated with stimulants as those born in September. Why? Because they were the youngest children in the class. This was estimated to account for about 900,000 inaccurate diagnoses, and studies in

Canada and Iceland confirmed the pattern. What this indicates is failure to distinguish ADHD from simple immaturity.

Another study, described in the book *The ADHD Explosion,* showed that the rate of ADHD skyrocketed in locations where "No Child Left Behind" and similar programs were put in place. Under these programs, all students must take standardized tests, the results of which determine school eligibility for certain federal funds. If schools do not qualify, penalties can result, including the firing of administration and staff. It seems that when teachers and schools depend on test results for their economic survival, diagnosing and medicating children to perform better becomes an attractive option.

The great variability in ADHD prevalence from state to state is further evidence of the capriciousness of diagnosing. For example, in 2011 the ADHD rate in Indiana was 13.8 percent, almost double that of neighboring Illinois, where it was 7 percent. Similar disparities exist between adjoining counties with similar populations.

The two most prominent reasons for overdiagnosis of ADHD are (1) high demand for treatment from teachers, schools, and parents, all under great pressure for children to perform, and (2) inadequate and rushed evaluations by physicians and other providers lacking sufficient time to do them right. An ADHD evaluation should take into account all aspects of a child's life, including relationships with family, school, and community, as well as individual strengths and weaknesses. Many conditions can be mistaken for ADHD—among them, learning disabilities, anxiety, post-traumatic stress disorder (PTSD), and sleep apnea—and these will be missed without careful inquiry.

With a July birthday, Maya, it turned out, was one of the youngest children in her class. It was unclear if her ADHD symptoms really were making a significant impact in more than one area of life. Her school problems seemed highly dependent on which teacher she had. One study showed that of children who were rated by one teacher as having inattention symptoms of ADHD, fewer than 50 percent were so rated by their teacher in the following year.

Medications for ADHD

The most common medications used to treat ADHD are psychostimulants. Methylphenidate (Ritalin, Metadate, Concerta) is the best known of these. Others are dextroamphetamine/amphetamine (Adderall), lisdexamfetamine (Vyvanse), dexmethylphenidate (Focalin), and atomoxetine (Strattera). They all have a similar mode of action, expected benefits, dangers, and side effects.

These medications increase the availability of two important neurotransmitters, dopamine and norepinephrine, and stimulate the frontal lobe of the brain. The frontal lobe is responsible for executive function — the ability to plan, focus, and control impulses — which is exactly what is difficult for those with ADHD. When psychostimulants improve executive function, they also dramatically decrease hyperactivity.

Hundreds of short-term studies have shown that these medications are effective for about 70 percent of patients who actually have ADHD, both children and adults. They may enable children to sit still, focus better, learn more efficiently, and restrain impulsive behavior. For some, psychostimulants can be a real lifesaver.

The cost of ADHD drugs ranges from $15 to $500 a month. Even though children are still the primary users, in recent years the greatest increase in expenditure on them has been among adults.

THE PROBLEMS WITH PSYCHOSTIMULANTS

There are two serious problems with psychostimulants. First, these medications can have significant short- and long-term adverse effects. Second, there is no good evidence that they are of long-term benefit.

Following is a list of their more common side effects:

abdominal pain

agitation

anxiety

decreased appetite and weight loss

decreased growth

hallucinations

headaches

increased blood pressure (may be more of a
    problem in adults)

increased risk of substance abuse and addiction

tics

trouble sleeping

All the above are fairly common. Additionally, many children experience more subtle effects. They may do well, but parents say they "just don't seem to be themselves." Like Maya, they may lose their joy or spontaneity. Some become overtly depressed, irritable, or angry. Often they have periods of increased hyperactivity or irritability as the drug wears off in the late afternoon, sometimes necessitating the addition of more or different medications.

The issue of hallucinations is a serious one, probably more common than parents and doctors realize. Past studies found that 1 to 3 percent of children developed hallucinations while taking psychostimulants. A recent study showed that 62 percent of children of parents with a history of major depression, bipolar disorder, or schizophrenia developed psychotic symptoms while taking psychostimulants—a troubling finding.

Most of the side effects resolve when the medication is stopped, although tics may persist and growth may not catch up. Fortunately, most children revert to their normal selves quickly, just as Maya did.

Good long-term studies on psychostimulants for ADHD have been few and far between and have yielded disappointing results. The most famous of these was the so-called Multimodal Treatment of Attention Deficit Hyperactivity Disorder (MTA) study, performed by distinguished professors from several academic universities. They randomly assigned 564 children to four groups. The first group received medication only, the second medication and behavioral treatment, the third behavioral treatment only, and the fourth whatever treatment was offered by their community doctors. After one year, both medication groups did significantly better, a finding hailed by proponents of drug treatment. But by the second year, 50 percent of the benefit had disappeared, and by three years out there was no difference between the children who had taken medication and those who had not. To quote directly from the study: "The modest significant advantages we found at the twenty-four-month assessment for the MTA Medication Algorithm...were completely lost by thirty-six months. Likewise, we found no differences in rates of ADHD diagnosis and other comorbid conditions across the originally assigned treatment groups at thirty-six months." Bottom line: the children got better with or without medication.

Results of another long-term investigation, the Preschool Attention Deficit Hyperactivity Treatment Study (PATS), were similar. It followed 230 preschool children diagnosed with ADHD between ages three and five up to age ten. By age ten, 79 percent of those taking medication still had symptoms, as opposed to 73.1 percent of those not taking medication. The symptoms of those taking medication were just as severe as those not taking it.

Why do drugs that are initially effective fail to provide long-term benefit? It could be that the brain develops resistance to the effects, or that the medications are not managed optimally, or that so many children improve on their own that any benefits cannot be detected.

The last possibility is supported by research data. One study measured the thickness of the cerebral cortex in the frontal lobe of the brain as children grew. Those with ADHD had a three-year delay in the development of the frontal cortex, but many caught up as they matured. In fact, only 30 to 50 percent of children diagnosed with ADHD still fit ADHD criteria when they are adults. Therefore, we are treating many children who may be improving on their own.

If we cannot prove that psychostimulants are

effective in the long term, how concerned should we be about possible harm—in particular, their effects on the developing brain? There do not appear to be obvious long-term side effects. We have used these medications since the 1950s, and patients on them for years do not develop heart failure, kidney problems, or other major physiological problems. Nor do we see an increase in severe psychiatric problems like schizophrenia or major depression. An obvious concern is addiction, given the numbers of people who are dependent on stimulants. However, no one has been able to study the more subtle effects of these medications. Since psychostimulants modify neurotransmitter and brain function and the brain continues to develop into young adulthood, it is unreasonable to assume these medications would not affect that process. But no one really knows. We are doing a vast experiment on several million children, with results that are very difficult to predict.

The long-term studies that could give us answers are hard to do on children, but they have been done on rats, and the results should give us pause. Exposure to methylphenidate in adolescent rats is associated with persistent neurobehavioral consequences in later life. It makes them more sensitive to stress and more anxious—hardly changes we would like to see in our children.

The Cochrane Database of Systematic Reviews publishes evaluations of the effectiveness and safety of medical interventions. It is perhaps the most widely accepted medical authority on this subject. In 2015, Cochrane looked at the efficacy of methylphenidate for ADHD. The conclusions questioned the quality of evidence used to support its use, suggested that better studies were needed, and highlighted the "urgent need for large randomized controlled trials of non-pharmacological treatments."

A final concern is whether psychostimulants increase the likelihood that treated children will grow up to be substance abusers — an important question because the rate of substance abuse disorder in teenagers with ADHD is 10 percent, compared to 3 percent in the non-ADHD population. Available research data do not suggest any correlation, but the risk of abuse and addiction to psychostimulants in college students is a serious issue. These medications are illicitly available on all college campuses in our country. Some students use them just to get better grades, as previous generations may have used caffeine or diet pills; many use them to get high, often with grave consequences. In one survey, nearly two-thirds of students at a large mid-Atlantic university had been offered stimulant medication, and 31 percent admitted to abusing ADHD drugs. As quoted in one study, a young college student said, "You swallow Adderall to study and snort it for fun."

INTEGRATIVE MEDICINE APPROACHES TO MANAGING ADHD

Given the significant limitations of psychostimulants, how else can we manage patients diagnosed with ADHD who really do require treatment?

First and foremost, behavioral treatment of ADHD should always be recommended along with medication. This may involve parent training, direct behavioral therapy, and certain classroom modifications. Too often, behavioral treatment goes by the wayside once medication has begun. Changes in parenting style or in the school environment can be as effective as any drug for children with ADHD. (Recall that Maya did so well in one year and so poorly in the next; sometimes the fit between a student and the school or teacher can make all the difference.)

Integrative medicine can draw from a number of effective interventions with low risks of side effects. Diet, for one, can have a major influence on ADHD symptoms. Several studies have shown that many children with ADHD are "sensitive," although not truly allergic, to certain foods. When these foods are removed from the diet, symptoms improve. For example, a 2011 study published in the prestigious British medical journal the *Lancet* showed that 64 percent of children improved significantly when placed on an elimination diet. The most common offenders are gluten (in wheat and other grains) and casein (in cow's milk). Artificial colors and other additives can also worsen ADHD, as shown in several studies. In Europe this research is taken so seriously that a warning label is required on food products with certain artificial colors.

Deficiencies of iron and zinc have both been shown to correlate with ADHD. Omega-3 fatty acids, found primarily in fish, are generally deficient in affected children; supplementation with fish oil can be beneficial. Although there is only limited research on the microbiome and ADHD, one study did find that giving supplemental probiotics to infants significantly decreased their chances of developing ADHD.

A recent exciting option is the use of EEG neurofeedback, in which children use biofeedback methods to learn to modify their brain waves. Good research shows this to be effective, although expense is a major drawback. Other promising computer-aided techniques for improving cognition and concentration are in development.

Evaluating and correcting lifestyle issues is also very important, starting with sleep problems. Both sleep apnea and simple lack of sleep may be major contributors to the severity of ADHD. In fact, the amount of sleep a child gets can be a significant predictor of success in school. The same is true of exercise. Several studies have shown that exercise is of benefit for those with ADHD, and most of our children get far too little of it. More time spent in nature has also been linked to a decrease in ADHD symptoms.

Mind-body interventions like yoga and mindfulness training may help as well; ongoing studies are beginning to demonstrate their usefulness. And breath work can be an effective remedy for hyperactivity.

BOTTOM LINE

ADHD is highly overdiagnosed. Children with learning or behavioral difficulties should be carefully evaluated before being labeled with the disorder. For those who do have ADHD, medication can be a viable option but should be just one component of an integrative treatment plan. Medication treatment is warranted only if one of the following circumstances is true:

- The child is unable to learn.
- The ADHD is causing great difficulty in the home environment.
- The child is unable to make or keep friends due to the ADHD.
- The child's self-esteem is suffering because of any of the above problems.

Even in these circumstances it may be advisable to

try nondrug approaches first, because the long-term efficacy of psychostimulants for managing ADHD is questionable, and their safety in long-term use—especially in terms of brain development—is unknown. Furthermore, illicit methylphenidate and related stimulants are now major drugs of abuse and addiction.

12

Opioids and the Treatment of Chronic Pain

Pain is a universal human experience. Treatments and remedies for pain abound in folk medicine and traditional systems of healing, many of them effective, especially for acute pain. Most effective of all is the opium poppy *(Papaver somniferum)*, used in the Old World since ancient times. Derivatives of opium—from morphine and codeine to oxycodone (OxyContin)—collectively known as *opioids,* are still our most powerful analgesic drugs. They are quite safe when used appropriately, especially for short-term management of acute pain. But long-term use to treat chronic pain is another story. Overuse, misuse, and abuse of opioids are now rampant, harming individuals and society. According to figures from the Centers

for Disease Control, in 2010 American physicians prescribed enough of them to treat every adult in the
country around the clock for a month. In the political
campaigns leading up to the 2016 presidential election,
voters in many states, especially in New England, told
candidates that opioid abuse was their greatest concern,
more so than the economy or threats of terrorism.

Consider this case history:

Greg graduated high school with honors. Several years
later, in 2007, he decided to join the army, as many
members of his family had before him. During his initial fifteen-month tour in Iraq, which involved several
combat missions, he wrote to his girlfriend and parents
about his increasing battle with depression and frequent
nightmares. Shortly after returning home he was diagnosed with post-traumatic stress disorder (PTSD) and
received counseling for several months. After additional
training, Greg returned to Iraq for a second tour in
2010, serving as a medic for his unit in Baghdad.

During his time in Iraq he was involved in four impro-
vised explosive device (IED) attacks, suffering a painful shoulder injury as well as a concussion. (The
concussion was caused by an explosion that killed several members of his unit in the Humvee in front of
him.) Because his initial treatment with NSAIDs and
physical therapy did not significantly reduce his pain,
he began receiving daily opioids, including hydroco-
done combined with acetaminophen (Vicodin). In addi-

tion to his shoulder pain and nearly daily headaches, Greg was dealing with severe anxiety, insomnia, and nightmares. He also experienced significant weight gain and had recently been diagnosed with pre-diabetes. Subsequent to his discharge and evaluation at the local Veterans Administration (VA) hospital, he was diagnosed with mild traumatic brain injury (TBI). During a series of medical visits with different providers, his pain medications were escalated to long-acting morphine, oxycodone combined with acetaminophen (Percocet) as needed, plus alprazolam (Xanax) and zolpidem (Ambien).

Greg had hoped to find work in health care, but he was unable to hold a steady job. At one point, after being fired, he told his girlfriend that he was "ready to end it." She contacted his parents and siblings, who arranged to have him evaluated at a regional VA medical center with integrative medicine capabilities.

At his appointment, he discussed his feelings of failure and increasing thoughts of suicide. He also admitted to memory lapses and bouts of aggression that affected his relationships and ability to work. He confided that he was storing his opioid medication for the day that he could "no longer manage."

At this point a comprehensive plan of care was developed. Initially he was placed on a monitored detoxification program with behavioral counseling, including cognitive behavioral therapy. In addition, his team provided cranial therapy, acupuncture, and healing touch for pain relief as well as nutritional and exercise therapy to manage his weight and blood sugar. He also attended classes during his treatment, including a yoga program, tai chi, and vocational rehabilitation. After more than three months of intensive behavioral and integrative care he was able to return home, off all pain medication. He now relies on daily home exercise and biofeedback to keep his pain and anxiety under control. He has also been able to secure a job with a local nonprofit agency that helps homeless veterans with basic health care needs and housing.

THE NATURE OF CHRONIC PAIN

Pain can persist in the absence of the event that triggered it, developing into a stubborn, debilitating syndrome of chronic pain that resists treatment, undermines quality of life, and causes great frustration for patients, doctors, families, and society. The incidence of chronic pain syndrome has increased enormously in recent years, becoming a costly burden on the health care system and provoking much debate about treatment strategies. One reason for the increase is the number of returning war veterans with devastating injuries, many of which would have been fatal were it not for recent advances in trauma medicine. Poor treatment outcomes in this group, along with dependence on opioids, have drawn more attention to the difficulty of managing chronic pain. An emerging consensus is that medication alone cannot solve the problem.

Pain is the most common reason people see a doctor worldwide. It may start as an acute bout of low back, neck, or head pain. In most cases these episodes resolve, but for more than 1.5 billion people worldwide and more than 100 million Americans, the problem lasts more than several months, becoming chronic. Not only does pain at the initial site worsen with this transition, it becomes more likely to gradually transform into an entity that requires a completely different approach from the one we currently use. Chronic pain syndrome is also associated with trauma, migraine, arthritis, fibromyalgia, and neuropathy (nerve pain, a common complication of diabetes and adverse effect of some forms of cancer chemotherapy).

We now understand that as pain becomes chronic, brain areas that perceive it begin to change physically and to communicate with nearby areas in the brain that normally have nothing to do with pain. Involvement of these other regions appears to be related to difficult symptoms that often accompany chronic pain, such as fatigue, disturbed sleep, depression, anxiety, and cognitive impairment. These "comorbidities" greatly complicate the management of chronic pain, making it fundamentally different from acute pain. In many settings, unfortunately, patients with chronic pain syndrome are still treated as if they have acute pain.

The newer, integrative approach stresses individual-ized treatment and uses many different modalities coor-dinated by a team of health care professionals. Analgesic medication is a component of this approach but never the sole component or even the most important one.

NSAIDs and Acetaminophen

Aspirin and other nonsteroidal anti-inflammatory drugs (NSAIDs) are the most widely used analgesics, along with acetaminophen (Tylenol), also known as paracetamol, a different kind of medication that has little effect on inflammation. People commonly self-medicate with these drugs, and those with chronic pain syndrome may take them frequently over long periods of time.

NSAIDs are discussed in detail in chapter 8. They have significant potential for harm with long-term use as well as for interactions with other drugs, and they should never be stand-alone treatment for chronic pain.

Acetaminophen is comparable to aspirin in analge-sic efficacy. It is generally safe, although overdoses, which are not uncommon, can cause severe liver damage and liver failure. In fact, acetaminophen toxicity accounts for most cases of acute liver failure in the United States and other Western countries; many of these are seen in emergency rooms, many require hospitalization, and some result in death. People who drink alcohol regularly are at greater risk of overdose, as are recreational users of products that combine acetaminophen and opioids; many such prescription medications are diverted to the black market. Heavy drinkers and those with known liver disease should be cautious about relying on acetaminophen to manage chronic pain.

Opioids

For moderate to severe acute pain, opioids are the drugs of choice. Two natural constituents of opium—codeine and morphine—have been around for a long time.* Codeine is a weak analgesic, often combined with aspirin or acetaminophen, and also used as a cough suppressant. Morphine is a major analgesic medication; like other opioids it is much more potent when administered parenterally—that is, not by mouth but by injection into a muscle or vein. Over the years, chemists have tinkered with these molecules to produce dozens of semisynthetic and synthetic analogs, often in a vain attempt to separate the analgesic properties from the addictive ones. Heroin was released to the world in 1898 as a safe and effective cough suppressant and pain reliever

---

* Technically, the natural constituents of opium are known as *opiates;* the term *opioids* designates semisynthetic and synthetic derivatives of opiates.

with none of morphine's risk for dependence, which by then was well known,* and there have been many similar claims made for new opioids ever since. Recently, pharmaceutical manufacturers have made available long-acting forms of morphine (like MS Contin) and other opioids, such as fentanyl (Duragesic), hydromorphone (Dilaudid), and oxycodone (OxyContin).

Opioid drugs work by activating the same brain receptors that bind opioids made within the body. These natural or *endogenous opioids* include endorphins, which affect mood and pain perception and can be released by many triggers, including exercise and acupuncture. It just happens that molecules made by the opium poppy bind to those same receptors.

For acute pain that resists NSAIDs and acetaminophen, opioids are very effective. They also work well for some types of chronic pain but not so well for others. Many experts now agree that the risks associated with use of these drugs are likely to outweigh the benefits when they are used long term for most types of non-cancer pain, including headache, back, and neck pain. For chronic pain that is episodic, such as pain

---

* It is only by historical chance that heroin is classified in the United States as a drug with high potential for abuse and no therapeutic benefit. In fact, it is not fundamentally different from morphine, only a bit more potent, so that it gives equivalent pain relief in lower dosage. This can be an advantage in patients who cannot tolerate the nausea or itching that higher doses of morphine often cause. Heroin is used medically in the UK and other countries.

associated with migraine, fibromyalgia, and neuropathy, acetaminophen and NSAIDs are preferable to opioids. A 2006 epidemiological study concluded, "It is remarkable that opioid treatment of long-term/chronic non-cancer pain does not seem to fulfill any of the key outcome opioid treatment goals: pain relief, improved quality of life, and improved functional capacity."

THE PROBLEMS WITH OPIOIDS

Opioid overdose can cause fatal depression of respiration by direct action on the brain center that controls breathing. This is unlikely in patients taking them regularly for chronic pain, because tolerance to this effect develops rapidly. It is more likely when opioids are combined with sedative drugs. The combination of opioids and benzodiazepines ("benzos" — see chapter 9) is especially dangerous, quadrupling the risk of overdose. (Greg, in the case presented at the beginning of this chapter, was on several opioids and two benzos.)

Otherwise, the adverse effects of opioids are more sources of discomfort than threats to life. Most common are nausea and vomiting, itching, sweating, dizziness, drowsiness, and constipation. In the elderly, dizziness can increase the risk of falls. Constipation can be severe. Some people on long-term opioid treatment experience an odd intensification of sensitivity (*hyperalgesia*), making the lightest touch unbearable and the pain actually worse.

In end-of-life care—for example, of people with end-stage cancer who are experiencing constant pain—opioid analgesia may be a necessity, but the cognitive effects of the drugs, sometimes called "mental clouding," can be distressing for those who wish to remain lucid through the dying process and be able to communicate with loved ones. Some hospice physicians say that managing pain with opioids in this setting is challenging, and that it takes skill and art to provide adequate analgesia without diminished awareness.

Of course, the overriding concern about long-term use of opioids is addiction and its destructive effects on individual lives and on society. Regular use of any opioid analgesic can lead to tolerance (the need for higher doses to maintain a desired effect), physical dependence, and addiction. Physical dependence, marked by prominent withdrawal symptoms when an opioid is discontinued, is common but is not the same as an addiction disorder, which is much more serious. An estimated 5 percent of those who stay on opioids for more than a year develop addiction disorder. People who experience euphoria from opioids, especially when they first receive them by injection, are more at risk, as are those who rely on opioids to dampen psychological pain. (As noted earlier, psychological distress is a major component of chronic pain syndrome.) Addiction disorder represents derangement of the brain's reward system. It is characterized not only by physical dependence but by obsessive focus on the drug, behavior problems, impaired social functioning, and loss of productivity.

In the late 1980s and early 1990s, use of opioids increased dramatically. This followed a call by noted pain clinicians to not undertreat pain, including non-cancer-related pain. It was also spurred by the introduction of the long-acting forms mentioned above and their vigorous promotion by manufacturers. The US Food and Drug Administration found it necessary to issue warning letters to some of these manufacturers. For example, it told one company that its ads "omit and minimize the serious safety risks associated with OxyContin and promote it for uses beyond which [it has] been proven safe and effective."

Overall, opioid prescriptions have quadrupled since 1999, with a similar sharp increase in opioid-related overdoses, injuries, and deaths. As many as 60 percent of returning war veterans suffer from chronic pain (compared to about 30 percent of civilian Americans). And veterans are twice as likely to die from accidental opioid overdoses as non-veterans. Furthermore, there has been an alarming rise in prescription opioid abuse. Pharmaceutical companies produce vastly more of these drugs than are needed for legitimate medical use, and much of that production is diverted to the black market. OxyContin abuse is notorious; the drug is so popular in rural America that it has become known as "hillbilly heroin." Prescription opioid abuse and misuse cost the United States more than $60 billion each year, almost half of which is attributable to workplace costs (such as lost productivity) and half to health care costs (such as abuse treatment). Placing someone on opioids, such as OxyContin, costs by one recent estimate about $6,000 a year. This does not take into account the dollars spent on drug testing and monitoring, treatment of potential side effects, and drug rehabilitation when needed.

Doctors are to blame for most of this. Ever since morphine was isolated from opium, they have prescribed it and related drugs recklessly, often with little heed of the risks, convincing themselves and patients that each new opioid product is safer than the last. When doctors are called to account for their behavior, as happens periodically, they back away from using opioids, sometimes withholding them from patients who really need them. Sooner or later they return to the same irresponsible prescribing habits. Dr. Richard A. Friedman, a professor of clinical psychiatry and the director of the psychopharmacology clinic at the Weill Cornell Medical College, wrote in a *New York Times* editorial in 2015: "It is physicians who, in large part, unleashed the current opioid epidemic with their promiscuous use of these drugs; we have a large responsibility to end it."

By 2011, many of the clinicians involved in promoting increased opioid use were publicly acknowledging that there were significant problems with reliance on these drugs for long-term management of chronic pain. In response to the rapid rise in the misuse and abuse of prescription opioids, a number of states began to restrict their availability. The federal government took action as well, subjecting manufacturers to greater scrutiny, insisting on better formulations, and requiring education of doctors about safe prescribing. For some of those in pain this has resulted in undertreatment, if opioids were a mainstay and especially if other therapies are not readily available or affordable. For doctors, it has been the continuation of an uncomfortable ride over the last century. For both patients and doctors, this situation has advanced the development and acceptance of integrative approaches to managing chronic pain.

INTEGRATIVE MEDICINE APPROACH TO MANAGING CHRONIC PAIN

A recent review of more than twenty lower-back-pain studies concluded that when exercise, acupuncture, and manipulative therapies are added to standard drug treatment, there is greater improvement in pain and function. One example of how this finding is being put into practice is the Oregon Pain Management Commission's integrative initiative. Based on the costs and poor outcomes of a medication-focused approach, the state passed an initiative in 2016 to provide integrative therapies for chronic pain syndrome in addition to conventional care, including acupuncture, massage, manipulation, yoga, and supervised exercise and physical therapy. I hope that other states will follow Oregon's lead and that patients, families, and health care providers will use the emerging findings to implement treatment for chronic pain—and demand insurance coverage for it. The VA has also backed away from reliance on opioids to manage chronic pain syndrome and is now actively promoting comprehensive care that includes acupuncture, yoga, mindfulness meditation, and physical therapy.

The experience of pain includes both the primary sensation of it and the brain's interpretation of that sensation. Local anesthetics like procaine (Novocain) block the former; opioids act in the brain to modify interpretation of pain signals. With opioid-induced analgesia, a patient may report that "the pain is still there, but it doesn't bother me" or "it is as if the pain is happening to someone else." Under hypnosis people often make the same kinds of statements. In good subjects (those with high capacity for trance), hypnosis can induce analgesia as complete as that from any opioid—complete enough for dental procedures and even major surgery without anesthetic drugs. The mechanism for this remarkable effect might involve endogenous opioids; in any case, it demonstrates the potential of using the mind-body connection to change the experience of pain.

Apart from hypnosis, mind-body therapies useful in managing pain include visualization and guided imagery, biofeedback, breath work, meditation, and mindfulness training. An impressive body of evidence supports the efficacy of mindfulness to help patients better live with chronic pain. It allows them to focus awareness on the present moment, rather than dwell on past painful sensations or anticipate those to come. Mind-body medicine should be a major component of integrative pain management, whether or not analgesic medication is required. (In my opinion, the absence of these therapies from Oregon's integrative pain management initiative is a glaring omission.) Yoga and various forms of relaxation training, including group relaxation, can also be helpful.

Massage, manual, and manipulative therapies (such as that offered by chiropractors and osteopathic physicians) should be considered in any cases where muscle tension, poor posture, and structural abnormalities contribute to pain. Exercise has now been confirmed to be a powerful anti-inflammatory intervention, able to reduce markers of inflammation linked to pain. Acupuncture also has a significant analgesic effect that might be mediated by endorphins.

"Biostimulation" is an umbrella term for newer therapies to reduce pain that direct electrical, magnetic, light, and sound stimulation to areas of the body. One example is transcutaneous electrical nerve stimulation (TENS), which can relieve musculoskeletal pain; TENS devices for home use are available. Also available are brain stimulation devices that deliver electromagnetic energy to shift blood flow and reduce excitability of specific areas of the brain involved in chronic pain syndrome. At the present time most can be accessed only in medical settings, but people will soon be able to get devices for home use (such as transcranial direct-current stimulators, or tDCS).

Cognitive behavioral therapy (CBT) can help chronic pain patients identify and change patterns of thought that contribute to the problem.

Group support can be tremendously helpful. Many leading medical institutions, including Cleveland Clinic and Boston Medical Center, are successfully using group settings for treating chronic pain. Additionally, some interventions, such as mindfulness meditation, can be done through an online community, allowing access for those who may not live near a class.

Diet and supplementation can help in multiple ways to reduce pain. First, as pain becomes chronic it is well known that areas of the brain that control taste and satiety change along with those that control mood. As a result, nutrient deficiency is common in chronic pain syndrome and can be worsened by long-term use of analgesic medications. Nutrients often in need of repletion include vitamin D, magnesium, omega-3 fatty acids, and coenzyme Q10 (CoQ10). Not infrequently, such deficiencies are overlooked.

An anti-inflammatory diet, known to improve overall health and reduce disease risk, can lessen any inflammatory component of pain and reduce the need for medication. In addition to emphasizing plant-based foods, the diet includes anti-inflammatory herbs and spices, such as turmeric *(Curcuma longa)* and ginger *(Zingiber officinale)*.

If disturbed sleep is part of chronic pain syndrome, it must be corrected, not with additional medication but by identifying contributing factors (such as use of caffeine and other stimulants and noise or light in the bedroom) and paying careful attention to all aspects of sleep hygiene.

As medical cannabis has become legal, many patients report using it successfully to manage chronic pain, both on its own and in combination with opioids. The active components of this plant—cannabinoids—interact with opioid receptors and, at least in some individuals, make it possible to maintain the analgesic effect of opioid medications with lower doses and less frequent administration. Ongoing research is looking at which strains and preparations of cannabis are most effective for pain relief.

BOTTOM LINE

Chronic pain is fundamentally different from acute pain and cannot be managed successfully with medication alone. Opioid drugs have an important role in controlling pain in specific settings, but reliance on them to manage chronic pain syndrome can have devastating results, not only for patients but also for families and society at large.

If you or someone close to you suffers from chronic pain syndrome, it is critical to insist on an integrative treatment plan. The exact cause of the pain may not always matter as much as how that pain has affected the brain and mind-body functioning. Medication cannot address the complex psychosocial, occupational, and lifestyle dimensions of chronic pain, nor can it reverse the brain changes that underlie it.

Doctors should be supportive of this approach, as it is in line with current pain treatment guidelines. They may also help you connect with a nurse case manager, health coach, or other health care advocate who can assist you with access to non-pharmacological treatments.

13

Antihypertensive Drugs

Don is an easygoing sixty-six-year-old man who was brought to the emergency department because his son and daughter-in-law found him lying on the floor of his small apartment, too weak to stand on his own. Don has multiple health problems, including heart disease, high blood pressure, type 2 diabetes, an enlarged prostate, depression, and post-traumatic stress disorder (PTSD). He had just returned home after a short rehabilitation stay at a nursing home to recover from hip replacement surgery.

In the emergency department, Don received the "million-dollar workup." In addition to an array of laboratory tests that ruled out electrolyte imbalances and anemia, he had an electrocardiogram (EKG) and chest x-ray, both normal. He also had a CT scan of his brain, which was reassuringly negative. He was then seen by the stroke team, who felt a stroke was unlikely but suggested that he be admitted to the hospital so that he could be observed and have more imaging done if needed.

The initial plan proposed by the neurology consult team was to consider an MRI to rule out problems with the cerebellum, the part of the brain that helps with balance and sense of position. However, tight spaces trigger severe anxiety for Don, so he would have to be placed under anesthesia to have the MRI.

Fortunately, the staff took time to learn more about Don's medical history. His blood pressure was slightly elevated, in the 150/90 range, but Don mentioned that he had been too weak to take his blood pressure medications that morning. The team spoke with his primary care physician and learned she had just scaled back two of Don's four antihypertensive drugs because he was having dizziness and blood pressure measurements as low as 70/50.

Don's family thought that his medications were to blame for his weakness, especially tamsulosin (Flomax), the one his urologist had prescribed a few months ago for difficulty urinating related to his prostate enlargement. In fact, it is also used to lower blood pressure. The tamsulosin was stopped, and the dose of one of his antihypertensive drugs, lisinopril (Prinivil, Zestril), was lowered. The timing of his medicines was also modified.

When all was said and done, Don's dizziness vanished with the medication changes. He walked out of the hospital after a costly and stressful three-day stay, symptom-free and not needing to have an MRI under anesthesia. His doctors agreed that his symptoms and subsequent need for hospitalization were due entirely to the adverse effects of medications.

PREVENTING HIGH BLOOD PRESSURE: A MEDICAL REVOLUTION

In 2014, 32.5 percent of American adults had a diagnosis of high blood pressure, also known as hypertension. Hypertension is often referred to as the "silent killer," because it usually produces no symptoms but is, without a doubt, linked to increased risk of heart attack, stroke, and any number of other debilitating—and deadly—health problems. Research continues to indicate that careful blood pressure control markedly decreases risk.

Hypertension was first described as a disease in 1808, but it was not until 1896, when invention of the sphygmomanometer enabled doctors to measure blood pressure, that it caught their attention. In fact, detection and treatment of high blood pressure resulted in a dramatic shift in Western medical philosophy, motivating health care professionals to focus more on prevention in caring for their patients.

By the 1960s, it was widely understood that high blood pressure correlated with stroke risk. Additional research over the next few decades established a link between hypertension and cardiovascular disease in general. Diagnosis and treatment of hypertension is one reason for the dramatic decline in deaths due to heart attack that were epidemic in the mid-twentieth century. We now know that elevated blood pressure can also impair cognitive function, damage the kidneys, and contribute to erectile dysfunction, loss of vision, heart failure, and the rupture of aneurysms (distended arteries).

In industrialized societies like ours, blood pressure rises with age in most people. Age-related hypertension is associated with stiffening of arteries and is so common as to be considered a normal consequence of growing older. But it does not exist in the few remaining hunter-gatherer societies, suggesting that it is more related to lifestyle than to the aging process. Key lifestyle factors are likely to be diet, physical activity, and stress. Our high consumption of processed and manufactured foods loaded with sodium and quick-digesting carbohydrates is far from the more natural whole-foods diet of hunter-gatherers and probably affects blood pressure for the worse. Regular physical activity keeps arteries more elastic and helps maintain normal weight, both of which correlate with normal blood pressure. And, while hunter-gatherers are not free from stress and anxiety, we seem to experience more of it.

The connection between stress and blood pressure is the autonomic nervous system, which regulates the tone of the smooth (involuntary) muscle that lines the walls of arteries. The sympathetic branch of that system constricts arteries, increasing blood pressure, while the parasympathetic branch relaxes them, lowering pressure. In the fight-or-flight response, sympathetic activity ensures a constant flow of blood to the brain by raising blood pressure. Many people in our population suffer from chronic overactivity of the sympathetic nervous system, as if it were reacting to an emergency that never ends, and this is surely one root of hypertension. The act of measuring blood pressure by a doctor or a nurse often creates anxiety and increases sympathetic nervous tone, distorting readings taken in a medical setting. Such "white-coat hypertension" may not give an accurate picture of a patient's average pressures. Nevertheless, doctors often prescribe antihypertensive drugs on the basis of such readings.

Quick Fixes: The Rise of Antihypertensive Drugs

There is little doubt that blood pressure should be neither too high nor too low. Recent research findings suggest that it is desirable to lower pressures that are even slightly above the 120/80 previously considered normal for most adults.* Drugs have now displaced all other therapies. In 2010, the United States spent nearly $42.9 billion on the management of hypertension. Some $20.4 billion of that was for medications, $13.0 billion for ambulatory visits, and the rest for emergency department care, inpatient stays, and home health visits. It costs the average American adult with hypertension more than $733 per year to manage it, when costs of medications, doctor visits, and various tests are taken into account.

That said, the most commonly used blood pressure medications are relatively cheap, at least compared to other classes of drugs. Most have been on the market for some time and are available in less expensive generic forms. In fact, a number of them are on the formularies of national pharmacy chains and cost just $4 a month. The question is whether or not that increased

---

* The upper number is the *systolic pressure*, or the maximum reached when the heart is fully contracted; the bottom number, or *diastolic pressure*, is the minimum when the heart is fully relaxed.

availability serves patients' best interests. The patient in the example above suffered harm because he was given too many medications at once that affect blood pressure.

How Blood Pressure Medicines Work — and the Problems with Them

Because adequate blood flow is vitally important for nearly all functions, the body regulates it carefully with complex nervous and hormonal mechanisms. The various antihypertensive drugs influence these mechanisms in different ways. For example, beta blockers work on the nervous system, while angiotensin-converting enzyme (ACE) inhibitors alter hormonal pathways. Calcium channel blockers relax the smooth muscle that lines blood vessels, and diuretics decrease blood volume by increasing urinary excretion of water. It is common today to treat hypertension by combining multiple medications with different mechanisms of action for a more powerful effect.

Any medication that lowers blood pressure can result in pressure that is too low, especially when used in drug combinations, as was the case with Don. Note that drugs used to treat other problems, like the tamsulosin Don was taking for his prostate-related urinary difficulty, can also lower blood pressure. While there is not a specific number used as a cut-off for dangerously low pressure in older adults, most doctors become concerned when the upper number dips below 100. With very low pressure, blood flow to vital organs like the brain and heart is inadequate, a potentially deadly condition known as "shock."

Many different classes of medications are used to control hypertension. Here are the most important ones and the adverse effects they can cause.

Thiazide Diuretics ("Water Pills")

These drugs came into use in 1958. Hydrochlorothiazide (HCTZ, Microzide) and chlorthalidone (Thalitone) are two examples. They reduce the amount of salt and water the kidneys reabsorb from urine, increasing urination and reducing blood volume. Side effects are dose related and tend to be rare: headache, weakness, upset stomach, itching, vision changes, and muscle cramps. Thiazide diuretics can also cause flare-ups in those with gout. People who take them complain about having to urinate frequently, but that is the intended effect. It is best to take these drugs in the morning rather than at bedtime.

Beta Blockers

First developed in 1973, dozens of these drugs are now in use. All block a specific type of receptor (the beta receptor) in the sympathetic nervous system, resulting in relaxation of the smooth muscle in arterial walls. Their generic names end in "-lol." Common examples are carvedilol (Coreg), atenolol (Tenormin), metoprolol (Lopressor, Toprol), and propranolol (Inderal). Beta blockers frequently cause fatigue, spasm of the airways (thus they should be used with caution in people with asthma), dizziness, erectile dysfunction, and low blood sugar. Metoprolol and propranolol, in particular, can cause insomnia and vivid dreams. Carvedilol can cause edema (retention of fluid in the lower extremities). Recent studies indicate that beta blockers are probably *not* the best first choice for blood pressure management in most people.

Alpha-2 Agonists

These drugs stimulate alpha-2 receptors in the nervous system, decreasing sympathetic tone. Many, but not all, have names that end with "-idine." The most common example of an alpha-2 agonist is clonidine (Catapres). All have a number of side effects, the most common of which are sedation, dry mouth, anxiety, constipation, nausea, and vomiting. They can also cause, more than other antihypertensive medications, a dramatic drop in blood pressure associated with changing position, such as when a person stands up after sitting (this is known as postural or orthostatic hypotension). Dizziness and fainting commonly result from postural hypotension.

Alpha-1 Blockers

Blocking alpha-1 receptors also lowers blood pressure. Most drugs in this class have names that end with "-osin," such as doxazosin (Cardura) and tamsulosin (Flomax). Like alpha-2 agonists, these drugs can cause orthostatic hypotension—a particular risk after a person takes the first dose of one of these medications. (These drugs also help manage prostate enlargement, which is why Don was put on tamsulosin.) Side effects include low heart rate, edema, dizziness, headache, fatigue, anxiety, and a variety of gastrointestinal and urinary effects, including increased urination. Alpha-1 blockers are not usually used as first-line blood pressure treatment.

Calcium Channel Blockers

In order to contract, muscle cells require that calcium ions move into them. Calcium channel blockers (CCBs) prevent calcium ions from moving into the muscle cells in arterial walls, thereby weakening their contractions. More relaxed blood vessel muscle translates into lower blood pressure. CCBs are considered first-line blood pressure drugs. The first CCBs, verapamil (Calan, Verelan, Covera-HS) and nifedipine (Procardia), were developed in 1977; amlodipine (Norvasc) is now widely used. CCBs work well for large blood vessel stiffness, which many elderly patients have. Side effects include constipation, nausea, dizziness, rash, swelling in the legs and feet, and drowsiness.

DRUGS THAT AFFECT THE RENIN-ANGIOTENSIN SYSTEM

The renin-angiotensin system (RAS) regulates blood pressure through hormonal mechanisms. When the kidneys sense that blood flow is decreased, they secrete an enzyme (renin) that increases blood levels of angiotensin I, an inactive precursor. Another enzyme (angiotensin-converting enzyme, or ACE), made by the lungs, acts to convert angiotensin I into angiotensin II, an active hormone that raises blood pressure by causing blood vessels to constrict. Drugs can interfere with this complex pathway in several different ways.

ACE Inhibitors

As their name suggests, these drugs prevent ACE from being released from the lungs, so it can't then turn angiotensin I into angiotensin II. The names of these drugs all end in "-pril": lisinopril (Prinivil, Zestril), enalapril (Vasotec), and captopril (Capoten). Like diuretics and CCBs, they are considered first-line blood pressure drugs, and they are particularly useful for people with diabetes because they also protect kidney function. (Kidney damage is a serious long-term complication of diabetes.)

Additionally, ACE inhibitors play a vital role in the treatment of heart failure. They can, however, cause a chronic, dry cough in 5 to 25 percent of people. They can also cause rash, diarrhea, drowsiness, headache, weakness, elevation in blood potassium levels, and abnormal taste sensation. A less common side effect is angioedema — swelling of the lips, mouth, and tongue that in some instances can be dangerous.

Angiotensin Receptor Blockers

Another way to decrease the effects of angiotensin II is by preventing it from binding to receptors in blood vessel walls. This is what angiotensin receptor blockers (ARBs) do. The names of these drugs end in "-sartan," such as losartan (Cozaar), candesartan (Atacand), and irbesartan (Avapro). They are often used when a person cannot tolerate an ACE inhibitor because of cough or angioedema; however, they can cause these same adverse effects, albeit less frequently. More common adverse reactions include first-dose postural low blood pressure, muscle cramping, insomnia, abnormal liver function, and lowered white blood cell counts.

Renin Inhibitors

First developed in 2000, drugs in this relatively new class bind to renin so that it can no longer act to produce angiotensin I. Aliskiren (Tekturna) is the main drug of this type. It should not be taken with an ACE inhibitor or an ARB, and its side effects are similar to those of both classes of drugs. It may also increase gout flares and the formation of kidney stones.

INTEGRATIVE MEDICINE APPROACHES TO LOWERING HIGH BLOOD PRESSURE

If you have been told you have high blood pressure, the first priority is to determine whether it is consistently elevated outside of a medical setting. The only way to do that is to monitor it yourself. Accurate, easy-to-use, reasonably priced digital blood pressure monitors are widely available. Get one and start recording your pressures several times a day at different times. You will find that they vary considerably. After a month or two, take the record to your doctor so that together you can decide whether treatment is necessary. As long as your blood pressure is not extremely high (that is, over 180/100) or associated with clear acute damage to vital organs, your goal should be to reduce it over the long term. Hypertension may be a silent killer, but it is also usually a very slow one. There is almost always time to experiment with lifestyle changes and other measures before starting on antihypertensive drugs. If these measures fail to bring your blood pressure down to the normal range and medication is necessary, ask your doctor to start with the lowest dose of the least powerful drug.

Using lifestyle measures and other therapies in combination with medication will often allow you to stay on lower doses of fewer drugs.

There are any number of ways to treat—and prevent—high blood pressure. Many of the methods described below will reduce the upper and lower blood pressure numbers by at least a few points each, and those benefits add up as you try several at a time.

Nutrition

Good evidence shows that both the dietary approaches to stop hypertension (DASH) diet and the Mediterranean diet can lower high blood pressure. Weight loss can make a big difference, too. Eating about 30 grams a day of fiber (at least 14 grams a day for every 1000 calories you eat in total) can also be helpful. (Note that it takes up to eight weeks for fiber to have its full effect.) People who eat more fruits and vegetables have lower risk of hypertension. And several recent studies indicate that eating unsalted nuts can lower blood pressure—especially pistachios, but other nuts as well; the effective dose is a handful a day.

Polyphenols, chemical compounds found in many plants, can also help. Cocoa and dark chocolate are good sources, as are grapes; that may be the reason why limited quantities of wine (red only, and just one glass a day or so, provided it does not lead to other health issues) have been found in some studies to reduce heart disease risk. Omega-3 fats, found in grass-fed animal meats, fatty cold-water fish, supplements, and other sources, also have benefit.

There seems to be a link between low vitamin D levels (under 30 ng/mL, especially) and higher blood pressure. Know your blood level of vitamin D and supplement appropriately.

For a long time, sodium has been associated with hypertension. A 2013 review found that reducing sodium from between 9 and 12 grams daily to between 5 and 6 grams daily has a significant beneficial effect; keeping it to 3 grams might be even better. The easiest way to do this is to reduce intake of processed and manufactured foods. Also, the effects of sodium are opposed by those of potassium, and you can increase your potassium intake simply by eating more fruits and vegetables. But keep in mind that a number of studies suggest, and a number of experts agree, that sodium is not as important an influence on blood pressure as we once thought.

Other Lifestyle Measures

A number of lifestyle factors favorably influence blood pressure. Physical activity, if done prudently, is good for practically all health issues, and hypertension is no exception. Yoga shows promise in what little research we have so far, as does tai chi. Adequate sleep is also important: we know that fewer hours of overall sleep at night and insomnia are tied to an increased risk of hypertension. Finally, quitting smoking is one of the best choices a person can make to improve blood pressure (and overall health). Every cigarette counts; cutting back even by one a day is of some benefit.

Relaxation and Social Connection

Relaxation training, such as breathing exercises, meditation, and biofeedback, lowers blood pressure by increasing activity of the parasympathetic nervous system. These approaches can drop the top blood pressure number by 10 and the bottom number by 7, if practiced regularly. Research indicates that people who are less isolated and more connected with others are less likely to be hypertensive.

Other Nondrug Therapies

A number of supplements have shown promise in lowering blood pressure—for example, hibiscus, coenzyme Q10, garlic, magnesium, and the amino acid L-arginine. Practitioners of Ayurveda and traditional Chinese medicine commonly treat people with hypertension and report success.

BOTTOM LINE

In treating high blood pressure, it is extremely important to take individual uniqueness into account. A doctor trained in integrative medicine will take a detailed history that may suggest ways to bring about more lasting improvements in health than simply depending on pills. How much is stress a contributor? Is there pent-up anger? Is a person living in a perpetual state of fight or flight? What about dietary habits? Or sleep quality? Is there a need to look for other physical contributors, such as the use of over-the-counter products and supplements that can raise blood pressure, particularly cold remedies and energy boosters that contain stimulant drugs (phenylephrine) and herbs (guaraná, ephedra)?

Remember that blood pressure is only one of many different risk factors for heart disease, stroke, and other serious health issues. Treating hypertension is important to these problems, but obesity, diabetes, tobacco dependence, depression, and any number of other contributors should be given attention as well. Medications cannot improve general health in the way that a tailored, thoughtful, and comprehensive treatment plan can. Integrative treatment can include medications but should not be limited to them.

14

Medications for Diabetes

Darla is a forty-two-year-old woman fighting for her life — but not in the way you might think. She's not tied to tubes and medication drips in an intensive care unit; instead, she's confined to a wheelchair.

Darla knows that it didn't have to turn out this way. As she gained weight into adulthood, her blood sugar crept up. When she was diagnosed with diabetes, she worried how it might affect her life — but not very seriously. She had a busy life with a stressful job, young children, and a strained marriage. Health was never her top priority. She was placed on one medication after another, but none of them turned things around. Some made her tired, while others caused weight gain or swelling. Most were expensive.

After the last oral medication failed to control her

diabetes, she was prescribed insulin. The syringes and vials were hard to manage, as was remembering when to inject herself. She tried, she really tried, but things got worse. She suffered severe damage to the joints of her feet (Charcot joints), caused by repetitive trauma associated with loss of sensation due to uncontrolled blood sugars. The only effective treatment was complete rest. Previously full of energy and accustomed to running around chasing her kids, she was told to stay in a wheelchair for three months, then six, then for an indeterminate amount of time.

One afternoon, just after turning forty, she experienced pressure in her chest. She brought her kids to their activities and completed an errand or two—but something was definitely wrong. At the hospital emergency department, she was told she was having a heart attack and was whisked into the cardiac catheterization ("cath") lab to have lifesaving stents placed in her heart. When she left the hospital, four new medications were added to her list.

She desperately wanted to walk again and was highly motivated to turn her diabetes around. By now, she was on whopping doses of insulin, which made her tired and packed on even more pounds. With each visit, she was told to take more insulin, even though her numbers improved only slightly. She wondered where it all had gone so wrong and what she could have done differently.

What Is Diabetes?

Diabetes mellitus,* a condition of elevated blood sugar with multiple metabolic consequences, has been recognized for centuries. Central to diabetes are problems with insulin, a hormone made by the pancreas that controls the transport and metabolism of sugar in the blood and throughout the body. Modern medicine recognizes two types of diabetes. In type 1, an autoimmune disease formerly called "juvenile diabetes," there is a deficiency of insulin; regular injections of the hormone are lifesaving and necessary.

In the much more common type 2 diabetes, resistance to the effect of insulin develops in genetically predisposed people—there are many of them—in response to eating too much of the wrong kinds of food and being sedentary. Several strategies are available to temper, reverse, and even cure the condition. When detected and managed early, especially in the so-called pre-diabetes stage, type 2 diabetes is best managed by modifications of lifestyle that focus on diet, exercise, and stress management. Unfortunately, the vast majority of

---

* The term comes from Greek roots and means increased flow of sweet urine, as opposed to the unrelated and much rarer condition, diabetes insipidus, in which the increased flow of urine is tasteless. Diabetes insipidus has nothing to do with insulin; it results from deficiency of a pituitary hormone.

type 2 diabetics don't even know they are at risk until the disease is more advanced and medications are necessary.

It's no exaggeration to say that type 2 diabetes is now epidemic in our population. Its incidence has increased fourfold over the last thirty years, now affecting one in four US adults over age sixty-five. Worldwide prevalence was 171 million in 2000, and the World Health Organization predicts that number will increase to 366 million by 2030. The cost of diabetes in 2007 was estimated at $174 billion and growing. If you don't now know somebody with type 2 diabetes, you probably soon will.

Diabetes is an enormous burden for those who suffer from it and often for family members, too. It affects your entire life, often requiring medications that have to be taken several times a day and careful attention to what you're eating and how you are living. Worse, uncontrolled diabetes carries with it the possibilities of chronic pain, impaired ability to fight infections, blindness, heart disease, kidney failure, and other devastating complications.

For these reasons, medical providers take the management of diabetes seriously. Insurance companies and payers often tie clinicians' performance and reimbursement to how well they take care of their diabetic patients. Treatment plans are provided to doctors, nurses, and other health professionals to help optimize care. Diabetes progression and severity are measured in a number of ways, including monitoring signs and symptoms for complications. Much importance is placed on results of a blood test for hemoglobin A1C (HgbA1C), which reveals the average blood sugar over the preceding three months. For most patients, the target HgbA1C is below 7 percent; below 5.7 percent puts an individual into the normal range. Every 0.1 percent change in the HgbA1C is significant.

DIABETES MEDICATIONS — AND THE PROBLEMS WITH THEM

Upon diagnosis of diabetes the prescription pad will often come out before lifestyle modification is discussed. Here are some of the likely medications, with their benefits and downfalls.

Metformin

The first-line medication for most diabetics, and even pre-diabetics, is metformin (Glumetza, Glucophage). Alone in its class, this drug works by decreasing the production and release of sugar from the liver, a mechanism that protects us from having dangerously low blood sugar (hypoglycemia). Metformin also sensitizes tissues to respond better and more effectively to insulin. Since it does not directly increase insulin secretion, it is not associated with hypoglycemia, a risk with other diabetes medications. Its use is common and its cost relatively low.

Nearly everyone started on metformin experiences side effects, though rarely serious ones. Gastrointestinal upset, with mild discomfort and loose stools, almost always occurs at the start of therapy or with an increase in dose. This generally passes within several days. A rare but more serious side effect is lactic acidosis—the build-up of excess acid in the system. This is most likely to occur when kidney function is impaired or in the presence of a kidney toxin, such as the contrast agents used in CT scans and other imaging studies. For this reason, metformin is often discontinued when a patient enters the hospital. If it's restarted after discharge, gastrointestinal rumbling will probably return.

Many doctors are unaware that metformin causes vitamin B_{12} deficiency in almost a third of people who take it. Those prescribed this medication should have their levels of vitamin B_{12} checked regularly. Supplementation with vitamin B_{12} is a good idea for people taking metformin, especially since there is little potential for toxicity even with high doses.

Sulfonylureas

These medications work by pushing out more of the body's own insulin from the pancreas. A common side effect is hypoglycemia. Any increase in circulating insulin is also associated with weight gain. Sulfonylureas are widely prescribed and relatively inexpensive. Specific agents include glyburide (Micronase, DiaBeta, Glynase) and glipizide (Glucotrol).

But the sulfonylureas can be difficult to use. Besides causing weight gain, individual response to them is inconsistent. More serious is the possibility of pancreatic "burnout" resulting from the constant stress of being forced to release more and more insulin above physiologic demands. These drugs also interact profoundly with other blood-sugar-lowering medications (and herbs); both doctors and patients should be aware of those risks.

Thiazolidinediones

The thiazolidinediones (TZDs) are approved for both the prevention and treatment of diabetes. The two most prominent agents are rosiglitazone (Avandia) and pioglitazone (Actos). They work by increasing insulin sensitivity and decreasing circulating free fatty acids that have a direct effect on the metabolism of glucose. They were commonly prescribed in the past, until significant concerns about their adverse effects caused them to fall out of favor.

The saga of the TZDs is a cautionary tale. Soon after their release, they were associated with swelling in the legs and worsening of congestive heart failure, a serious condition in which the heart does not pump blood efficiently. Then an increased risk of bladder cancer was found in people on these medications.

There was more bad news to come. A 2007 summary of the known science on the safety of rosiglitazone stunned the medical community. Diabetics are at higher risk for heart disease than others, and this review paper indicated that taking rosiglitazone put patients at even higher risk of heart attacks. Given the gravity of this finding, doctors and patients alike backed away from using TZDs. In Europe, marketing of these medications was suspended by the European Medicines Agency, the equivalent of the US Food and Drug Administration. Subsequent reviews have suggested that this risk is lower than initially reported, but doubts persist, and use of rosiglitazone has plummeted.

Incretins

This group of medications is newer to the scene. They stimulate release of the body's own insulin, but only in response to intake of a high glycemic load—that is, meals high in quick-digesting starches or sugars. They also slow gastric emptying and decrease the release of glucagon, another pancreatic hormone that opposes insulin and raises blood sugar. Use is common, as providers have moved away from the pancreas-depleting sulfonylureas and the potentially toxic TZDs. Medications in this group include sitagliptin (Januvia), saxagliptin (Onglyza), exenatide (Byetta, Bydureon), and liraglutide (Victoza, Saxenda). All are costly, although many insurance companies now favor their use and have lowered copays.

The initial, primary side effect of these medications is weight loss—not unwelcome among commonly overweight or obese diabetics. Sound too good to be true? Of course, it is. The incretins also cause nausea and diarrhea, as well as hypoglycemia, particularly when paired with other blood-sugar-lowering agents. Of greater concern is pancreatitis, a potentially life-threatening inflammation of the pancreas. A possible link to pancreatic cancer has also been suggested, though proponents of the medications argue that diabetes itself increases that risk. Some of these agents have been associated with thyroid cancer in animal models.

Despite recognized adverse effects and risks, the incretins are the current favored medications in those who don't achieve adequate blood sugar control on metformin before going to insulin replacement.

Insulin

Insulin was isolated in the early twentieth century. Shortly thereafter, two scientists, Frederick Banting and John Macleod, won the Nobel Prize in Physiology or Medicine for their discovery of its therapeutic use in saving the lives of type 1 (insulin-deficient) diabetics; until that time, the diagnosis was universally fatal.

Insulin is now also commonly used to treat type 2

diabetes, if the medications described above fail to keep the condition in check. Its cost is variable, as it comes in many forms: ultra-long acting, long acting, regular, short acting, and ultra-short acting. Insulin must be injected or administered through a pump connected to a needle that remains in place throughout the day. It can be purchased over the counter in many states, though it more often requires a prescription. Typically, it is dosed to match the body's natural fluctuations of insulin secretion in response to eating and activity.

Patients who use insulin must monitor their blood sugar carefully throughout the day. Side effects include potentially severe, even deadly, hypoglycemia if dosed too high. All patients on insulin gain weight—ironically, this means that their requirement for the hormone increases. It's not uncommon for insulin-dependent diabetics to be caught in a perpetual cycle of insulin, weight gain, more insulin, more weight gain—leading to discouragement and frustration.

INTEGRATIVE MEDICINE APPROACHES TO MANAGING DIABETES

Given the downside of all the available drugs, many people with diabetes would prefer not taking medication and wonder if that is an option.

In fact, reversing type 2 diabetes is very possible—

if it is not too severe. Every person with diabetes should focus on a careful diet, one that limits concentrated sweets or sweeteners and is high in fiber and vegetables. Optimal weight should be the goal, as excess weight and obesity make control of blood sugar more difficult. Current nutritional advice is to follow a low-glycemic-load diet, which means avoiding foods that provoke a rapid, high spike in blood sugar after eating. This requires learning the glycemic values for various foods. (There are many books and online sources of information on glycemic index and glycemic load, including *The New Glucose Revolution for Diabetes* by Jennie Brand-Miller, MD, and health.harvard.edu/healthy-eating/glycemic_index_and_glycemic_load_for_100_foods.)

Regular physical activity is good for all of us and is especially important for people with diabetes. Not only does it help keep blood sugar in the normal range, but it also offsets the risk for some of the serious complications of the disease, particularly heart disease. The minimum goal is two and a half hours per week of moderate-intensity aerobic exercise, defined as being unable to freely carry on a conversation while you're doing it. Those not in the habit of exercising should start slowly, perhaps with the help of a trainer or health coach. It is good to complement aerobic activity with gentler forms of movement like tai chi and yoga.

Once diet and exercise are addressed, next steps might include the addition of supplements and botanicals known to lower blood sugar or mitigate diabetes complications. Some of the best studied and most promising include the following:

• Alpha-lipoic acid: While this supplement does not directly lower blood sugar, it helps restore insulin sensitivity and is effective in managing one common complication: peripheral neuropathy—the pain and numbness that develop most often in the feet and legs. Recommended dosing is 600 to 1200 milligrams daily.

• Capsaicin: A topical preparation of this compound, extracted from hot peppers, is also useful for neuropathy. It must be applied regularly four times daily.

• Berberine: Found in a number of plants (like the Oregon grape, *Mahonia aquifolium*), berberine improves blood sugar and retinopathy—the eye changes associated with diabetes that can lead to blindness. Take 200 to 300 milligrams two to four times daily after checking for drug interactions. Avoid in pregnancy.

• Chromium: This mineral can be used to lower blood sugar directly and reduce HgbA1C by an estimated 0.6 percent. The recommended dose is 1000 micrograms daily of chromium GTF. Avoid using higher doses, which can harm the kidneys and liver.

• Cinnamon: Known better as a culinary spice, this can be taken at concentrated doses of 1000 milligrams three times daily to lower blood sugar.

- Magnesium: One of the body's most prominent minerals, magnesium is often deficient in diabetics. Supplementation to correct low levels can lower blood pressure and blood sugar. Start with 300 to 600 milligrams daily of magnesium glycinate or magnesium chelate, which are less likely to cause loose stools.
- Bitter melon: Extracts of this unripe fruit *(Momordica charantia)*, much used in the cuisines of India, China, and southeast Asia, lower blood sugar.
- Prickly pear (*Opuntia* spp.): Extracts of both the fruit and pads of this cactus are used in Mexican folk medicine to treat diabetes; they have blood-sugar-lowering properties.

An integrative approach to diabetes includes stress management through such mind-body techniques as progressive muscle relaxation, guided imagery, mindfulness meditation, and hypnosis.

Traditional systems like Chinese medicine and Ayurveda also have much to offer for managing diabetes since it has been recognized as a disease for so long.

BOTTOM LINE

The impact of type 2 diabetes can be overwhelming. This is sad, considering how preventable the disease truly is. Our highly processed standard American diet and sedentary tendencies increase the likelihood that more and more people will develop it.

Medications for diabetes will always be needed, but they bring with them a burden of side effects and cost that could be avoided with appropriate changes in lifestyle. Our health care system and our society should encourage better lifestyle choices by making these choices more accessible and more affordable (as by subsidizing fruits and vegetables rather than commodity crops, for example). By changing diet, increasing physical activity, managing stress, and using natural remedies appropriately, most people with early and mild cases of type 2 diabetes can put the disease into complete remission, and many others will be able to keep their use of medications to a minimum.

15

Medications for Osteopenia and Other Preconditions

The "precondition" is a relatively new concept in medicine that has expanded marketing opportunities for Big Pharma and greatly increased the numbers of people taking medications. Diagnosis of preconditions is based on abnormal results of medical tests that supposedly predict the future development of a serious health condition unless treatment is started—with drugs, of course. Many people now take prescribed medications for pre-hypertension, pre-diabetes, and osteopenia (the newly minted term for "pre-osteoporosis"). But how legitimate are these diagnoses and the assumption that preconditions will inevitably progress without pharmacological intervention?

Cecilia's health problems began at age forty-two,

with the onset of premature menopause. Several years later, at age forty-seven, she had a bone scan that revealed low bone mass and a diagnosis of osteopenia, the condition of bone thinning that sometimes precedes osteoporosis. People with osteoporosis have an increased risk of fractures of the hip, wrists, and spine. While Cecilia's bones were not as fragile as osteoporotic ones, they were below average in density. Her doctor at the time advised her to stay on hormone replacement therapy to prevent further bone loss. A couple of years later, however, she was taken off the hormones when evidence from the Women's Health Initiative showed increased risks of disease from this therapy.

Her doctor switched her to alendronate (Fosamax), a drug in a class known as bisphosphonates. It did reduce further bone loss, but a few years later, after gaining weight, Cecilia ran into problems. At first it was only occasional nausea. But over time, despite taking the medication as directed with a full glass of water and waiting more than thirty minutes in an upright position before eating breakfast, she began to experience constant nausea and heartburn. The burning sensation behind Cecilia's breastbone did not resolve with less frequent dosing or taking over-the-counter antacids or acid-blocking medications. She was switched to a different bisphosphonate drug, but her symptoms continued to worsen. At last, an endoscopic procedure revealed inflammation and ulcers in her esophagus. Cecilia stopped the bisphosphonate to allow her esophagus to heal. At this point she was advised to try a different medication for her osteopenia, either raloxifene (Evista) or an intravenous bisphosphonate. When she learned that these drugs, too, posed serious health risks, she consulted an integrative family physician to discuss non-drug alternatives.

The new doctor looked for the underlying causes of Cecilia's bone loss. It turned out that her levels of magnesium and vitamin D were very low and she was not consuming enough dietary calcium. She was advised to eat more leafy greens, nuts, beans, whole soy foods (soy milk, soy nuts, edamame, tofu, tempeh), yogurt, and high-quality cheese. After supplementation with magnesium and vitamin D, her nutrient levels were restored to normal. She reduced her wine consumption, since drinking more than two glasses a day can harm bone health in women. And she began a program of weight-bearing and resistance exercises. Her bone scan stabilized in subsequent months and to date has not shown progression to osteoporosis.

COMMON PRECONDITIONS TREATED WITH DRUGS

An important aspect of Cecilia's story is that osteopenia is not an actual disease; it is a precondition. Osteopenia is defined by the World Health Organization as bone mass density between 1.0 and 2.5 standard deviations below the average for a young adult population (between ages eighteen and thirty-five). The measurements are usually taken at the hip and spine using dual-energy x-ray absorptiometry, known as DEXA or DXA scanning. Based on this definition, more than half of women and a third of men over age fifty in the United States are believed to have osteopenia.

People with osteopenia may or may not have further bone loss and develop osteoporosis, an actual disease characterized by very low bone mass — more than 2.5 standard deviations below the young-adult norm. The more than 10 million Americans with osteoporosis have fragile bones susceptible to fractures that lead to disabling pain, shrinking stature, and a higher rate of premature death.

Both osteopenia and osteoporosis are defined by bone mass density, which indicates the mineral content of bone. But the risk of actually suffering a fracture is determined not only by mineral content but also by a bone's strength, elasticity, and other factors. A more relevant measurement is the Fracture Risk Assessment Tool, or FRAX (shef.ac.uk/frax), created by the World Health Organization to measure a person's ten-year fracture risk. Besides bone mass density, it takes into account age, gender, weight, family history, smoking, alcohol, medications, history of previous fracture, and other health conditions.

Unlike people with osteoporosis, those with osteopenia usually have a FRAX score that indicates low fracture risk and often have no evidence of progressive bone loss. Yet, they are commonly started on strong drugs with potentially serious side effects. Why? That's a good question, especially since much safer and fully effective alternatives exist.

And osteopenia is not unique.

Strong drugs are also commonly used as first-line treatments for a number of other preconditions. The list includes pre-hypertension, a condition of borderline high blood pressure now identified in one in three US adults, which is often first treated with antihypertensive medications, and pre-diabetes, which affects 79 million Americans with blood sugar levels that are higher than normal, though not as high as in diabetes. Even mild cognitive impairment—thought of as a sort of pre-Alzheimer's disease—is now cause for drug therapy. Once again, we have to ask: Are we overmedicating?

To answer this question, let's take an in-depth look at the medicines used to treat osteopenia. The drugs prescribed for pre-hypertension and pre-diabetes are much the same as those used to treat hypertension and diabetes, which have already been described in detail in chapters 13 and 14. I will touch back on treatments for pre-hypertension and pre-diabetes in the final two sections of this chapter.

TREATING OSTEOPENIA WITH BISPHOSPHONATES

Several medications are prescribed to treat osteopenia and prevent osteoporosis. The bisphosphonates are considered effective first-line therapy and are far and away the most commonly recommended medications for osteopenia. Other drugs approved by the US Food and Drug Administration include the selective estrogen receptor modulators as well as estrogen itself.

Bisphosphonates were first synthesized in the late 1800s. Initially, they were used industrially to manufacture textiles, soften water, and prevent the formation of calcium deposits in water systems. They did not come into widespread use as medical drugs until the 1960s, when scientists studied one of them — etidronate (Didronel) — to see if it would prevent dental plaque. While it was never widely used for this purpose, other medical uses were soon discovered. Research showed bisphosphonates to be effective for a number of bone diseases, and they came into use as treatment for Paget's disease, multiple myeloma, and metastatic bone cancers. In the mid-1980s, they were tested as therapy for osteoporosis in postmenopausal women and were found to increase bone density and reduce fracture risk in these patients. As additional bisphosphonate drugs were developed, their use expanded to include men with osteoporosis, patients with high blood calcium, and those receiving bone-thinning corticosteroid medications. Today the drugs are also given to children with inherited skeletal disorders, such as osteogenesis imperfecta.

What all these conditions have in common is excessive bone breakdown. Our bones contain specialized cells called osteoblasts that build new bone, and others called osteoclasts that break down and resorb old bone so that new can be formed. For optimum bone health, the activity of osteoblasts must be in balance with that of osteoclasts. Decades of research have shown that bisphosphonates act in the body as anti-resorptive agents. In patients with excessive bone resorption, they act to inhibit osteoclast activity by attaching to binding sites on bone. When the body tries to break down bone containing the drug, the bisphosphonate seeps out and impairs the ability of the osteoclasts to continue bone resorption.

Bisphosphonates are now prescribed extensively as first-line agents to treat osteopenia and osteoporosis. Alendronate (Fosamax) and risedronate (Actonel) — when taken by mouth daily, weekly, or monthly — have been shown to decrease hip and spine fractures in numerous studies. In contrast, ibandronate (Boniva), when taken by mouth daily or monthly or given intravenously every three months, reduces fractures of the spine only. Another bisphosphonate, zoledronic acid (Zometa), is given intravenously every one to two years for the prevention of hip and spine fractures. The cost ranges from $600 to $2,400 a year for oral medications and $1,000 to $2,000 a year for intravenous medications.

The Problems with Bisphosphonates

Side effects are a big issue with these drugs. Gastrointestinal problems, such as nausea, abdominal pain, indigestion, heartburn, and esophageal inflammation or ulcers, occur frequently in patients taking oral bisphosphonates. To avoid adverse effects, the drugs must be taken with a full glass of water on an empty stomach, and the patient must not lie down or consume anything else for thirty minutes. The medications are sometimes given weekly or monthly, or in intravenous form, to help lessen these problems. Other potential side effects include low blood calcium, kidney problems, and blurred vision or eye pain. Bone or muscle pain may occur and does not always go away. In addition, some people get fever and flu-like symptoms for several days after receiving intravenous bisphosphonates. The drugs have also been linked to a possible increased risk for esophageal cancer and atrial fibrillation, an abnormal heart rhythm.

Among the many adverse reactions to the drugs are atypical fractures of the thigh bones. Yes, that's right: the bisphosphonates can cause the very fractures they're meant to prevent. How does this happen? Studies show that long-term bisphosphonate therapy can lead to reduced bone formation and "frozen bone." Normally, bone formation is linked in the body to bone resorption. So anything that decreases bone resorption can also inhibit bone formation. This is the case with the bisphosphonates: they reduce bone resorption but simultaneously decrease bone formation as a side effect. The bone can no longer repair itself properly and becomes damaged and weakened, with increased brittleness and a higher risk for fractures. These fractures usually run horizontally across the thighbones in areas of thickened cortical bone (the outer layer of bone)—a characteristic pattern found in bisphosphonate-induced fractures and not seen in other fracture types. Delayed healing or non-healing of the atypical fractures often occurs and frequently requires surgical treatment.

The "frozen bone" scenario described above may also lead to a truly frightening condition: osteonecrosis of the jaw, in which part of the bone in the mouth starts to die—with subsequent pain, swelling, and possible infection and fracture of the jaw. These stubborn problems tend to resist treatment. While the incidence of this devastating complication is low in people on oral bisphosphonate therapy, it can occur in up to 10 percent of patients with cancer treated with long-term, high-dose intravenous bisphosphonates. Other factors that increase the risk for developing osteonecrosis of the jaw include dental disease, dental extractions and implants, poorly fitting dentures, corticosteroid medications, and smoking.

In light of these potentially serious side effects, many authorities recommend limiting bisphosphonate therapy to three to five years. After taking a drug holiday, some people are restarted on the drugs. With anyone on a bisphosphonate, it's important to watch for drug interactions. Bisphosphonates can interact adversely with many prescription medications; multivitamins; supplements containing calcium, magnesium, or iron; as well as many foods and beverages.

Finally, the concept of "number needed to treat" is revealing. It refers to the number of patients needed to receive a treatment for a fixed time to achieve a particular outcome. When comparing strategies for fracture prevention, the number of osteoporotic patients needed to receive treatment for three years to prevent one hip fracture is forty-five for vitamin D, forty-eight for strontium ranelate, and ninety-one for bisphosphonates. A lower score means a more effective treatment. For managing the precondition osteopenia with bisphosphonates, the number needed to treat is very high, meaning the drugs are not very effective.

OTHER PHARMACEUTICALS FOR OSTEOPENIA

Besides bisphosphonates, a few other drugs are prescribed for osteopenia. The selective estrogen receptor modulators reduce the risk of spine fractures but not hip fractures. The most commonly used drug in this class, oral raloxifene (Evista), has hormone-like effects that reduce bone loss. It has the additional benefit of reducing a woman's risk for breast cancer. Side effects include hot flashes, blood clots, and an increased risk of stroke. Raloxifene's cost is similar to that of oral bisphosphonates. Another medication prescribed for many years to prevent osteoporosis is the female hormone estrogen. While estrogen reduces the risk of hip and spine fractures, research from the Women's Health Initiative found that the hormone's harms—particularly the increased risk for blood clots and stroke—exceed its benefits. As a result, many physicians do not prescribe estrogen for osteopenia alone; they might use it only if a woman has additional menopausal symptoms such as hot flashes. When hormones are advised, the transdermal application of bioidentical products (those with the same chemical structures as the body's own hormones) may cause fewer side effects and have a somewhat lower risk profile than other forms of estrogen.

INTEGRATIVE MEDICINE APPROACHES TO TREATING OSTEOPENIA

Since osteopenia precedes any real disease and may not lead to further bone loss, doctors trained in integrative medicine don't automatically turn to drugs initially. A number of options, including lifestyle measures and dietary supplements, provide effective means for preventing progression to osteoporosis.

A balanced diet is key to avoiding bone loss. Aim for at least four to five servings of vegetables and three to four servings of fruit each day. Produce is packed with bone-boosting nutrients like calcium, magnesium, potassium, and vitamins B, C, and K. Your bones also need adequate protein for skeletal strength and repair. That can come from a combination of animal sources like poultry, eggs, dairy products, fish, and lean meat as well as vegetable sources like soy foods, other legumes, nuts, seeds, and whole grains. Whole soy foods have a well-known beneficial effect on bone density.

Calcium is an important mineral for bone health; a deficiency may accelerate bone loss. Try to get the calcium you need from food if possible. The best sources are dairy products, leafy greens, seaweed, fish canned with the bones, nuts, seeds, and beans. Consult with your physician before taking dietary supplements. Calcium citrate is the best-absorbed form, especially in older people and those with low stomach acid or on acid-blocking drugs. Blood levels of vitamin D must be optimal in order to absorb and use dietary calcium efficiently.

Don't forget about magnesium. This mineral is a major constituent of bone, yet most people don't get enough. Trace minerals such as boron, zinc, manganese, selenium, and silicon also play vital roles in bone health. You can get them by eating leafy greens, whole grains, nuts, seeds, and beans as well as by taking supplements. Research indicates that the trace element strontium stimulates bone formation and is effective for preventing bone loss. The most-studied form, strontium ranelate, has been linked to a small increased risk for cardiovascular disease. It is not available in the United States, but other forms of strontium are — though they have not been studied for safety or efficacy.

Several vitamins are often low in people with osteopenia. Vitamin C in citrus and tomatoes helps make the protein collagen that provides the framework for bone. Many studies have documented the key role vitamin D plays in bone health. Adequate amounts are essential for calcium absorption through the intestinal wall. The micronutrient also helps prevent falls in seniors provided it is not taken in excessively high doses. Blood testing is the best way to check your vitamin D status. If it's deficient, ask your physician if you need supplemental vitamin D_3, also known as cholecalciferol. Sun exposure without sunscreen for fifteen minutes daily will supply some cholecalciferol. Vitamin K_2 (menaquinone) directs calcium to stay out of your arteries and go into your bones. While our gut microbes make some vitamin K_2, production falls as we age. The best sources are fermented dairy and whole soy products as well as dietary supplements.

Besides good nutrition, your bones need physical activity. Research shows that weight-bearing exercises like walking are effective for increasing bone density of the hips and spine. Resistance exercises such as weight lifting or calisthenics also stimulate bone building. Removing home hazards and doing balance activities, like tai chi, yoga, or simply standing on one foot, can help reduce the likelihood of falls.

In addition, pay attention to bone-sapping toxins in your home and environment. Tobacco smoke is the number one culprit. If you smoke, talk to your physician about how to quit. Excess alcohol is also very hard on bones. Women who consume more than two drinks a day and men who imbibe more than four have an increased risk for osteoporotic fractures. Caffeinated beverages are another challenge. Drinking more than two and a half cups of coffee or five cups of tea each day may increase risk. Last but not least are prescription medications. Speak to your physician about alternatives if you take any drugs known to promote bone loss. Common ones are corticosteroids, phenytoin (Dilantin), lithium, proton pump inhibitors (PPIs), tamoxifen (Nolvadex), and excess thyroid hormone.

INTEGRATIVE MEDICINE APPROACHES TO TREATING OTHER PRECONDITIONS

Integrative medicine offers solutions for preconditions besides osteopenia. For pre-hypertension, a condition of borderline high blood pressure that affects millions of Americans, weight loss and moderate exercise along with dietary modification, relaxation techniques, and specific supplements can help. In patients with pre-diabetes, blood sugar levels are higher than normal but not as high as in diabetes. Research shows that diet and exercise are twice as effective as the drug metformin (Glucophage, Glumetza) for reducing the progression of pre-diabetes to diabetes (a 58 percent reduction with lifestyle change compared to 31 percent for the drug). Dietary supplements such as chromium, magnesium, berberine, and alpha-lipoic acid may be beneficial, as may blood-sugar-lowering herbs like bitter melon and prickly pear. For details on integrative treatments for these preconditions, please see chapters 13 and 14.

BOTTOM LINE

Our health care system has a pill for every ill. Drugs are prescribed for full-blown diseases as well as for conditions that are not yet diseases but might, or might not, someday become them. Drug companies have widely promoted the idea of preconditions to patients and doctors alike to sell more drugs.

Most people with osteopenia have a FRAX score that indicates a low fracture risk. They do not need drug therapy, since the risk outweighs the benefit. I consider preventive drugs only for osteopenic people with the greatest fracture risk—such as those with very high FRAX scores or a history of previous fractures.

Last but not least, diagnosing people with a precondition can cause needless worry. I see many patients who are stressed about their "osteopenia" or "prediabetes," when they could more productively focus on improving their health. For help reaching wellness goals, I advise partnering with a physician trained in prevention. Keep in mind that getting diagnosed with a precondition does not mean you are destined to develop a condition requiring lifelong drug treatment. Most people with preconditions can successfully modify or reverse them by means of simple lifestyle measures.

16

Overmedication of Children

An estimated 263.6 million prescriptions were written for children and adolescents in the United States in 2010. Let me recount the case histories of two young patients that illustrate the pitfalls of this kind of overmedication.

Kim

Kim is a two-year-old brought to the pediatric emergency department by her grandmother. The toddler had been agitated and crying inconsolably for the past six hours, and the grandmother was at her wit's end. Kim's parents left on a trip that morning and were unreachable. There was no history of trauma or abuse and no time that day when she had been out of her grandmother's care. Kim was finishing a course of amoxicillin for an upper respiratory illness (URI) but was an otherwise healthy child. Physical exam was normal except for extreme agitation. Results of blood tests, x-rays, and a brain scan were also all normal, as was a spinal tap performed to rule out serious infection or trauma. But results of a urine toxicology screen came back positive for four chemicals: guaifenesin (an expectorant), dextromethorphan (a cough suppressant), phenylephrine (a stimulant and decongestant), and acetaminophen (Tylenol). You can read about the shortcomings and dangers of these drugs in chapter 5. As it turned out, Kim's parents had given her a generous dose of an over-the-counter (OTC) cough and cold medicine before dropping her off. The child was admitted to the pediatric unit for observation due to accidental overdose and hyperstimulation from the OTC medication. She remained agitated for a total of twenty-four hours before symptoms resolved.

OVERMEDICATING CHILDREN WITH COLD MEDICINES

Each of the drugs found in Kim's system is a common ingredient in OTC cough and cold medicines. These products generally contain mixtures of drugs, alcohol, sugars, and artificial dyes and account for millions of dollars of annual sales for use in children. They remain very popular despite the fact that this class of drugs was voluntarily withdrawn from the market in 2007 for use in children under age two because of serious safety concerns. Although the US Food and Drug Administration and the American Academy of Pediatrics (AAP) have advised against giving them to children under age six, studies show that use in the two- to six-year-old age group has actually increased.

Parents typically reach for these medications to relieve a stuffy nose, calm a cough, and reduce a fever. Easy availability and colorful displays on drugstore shelves suggest safety. Nonetheless, the 2012 annual report of the American Association of Poison Control Centers lists OTC cough-cold medications among the top three products associated with fatality in children under age five.

The frequency of head colds in children and the potential toxicity of the OTC drugs commonly used in their treatment should motivate us to explore non-pharmacologic alternatives. We should first be informed about the ingredients in the OTC cough-cold products. As noted in chapter 5, guaifenesin is ineffective; large randomized studies have shown it to have no measurable effect. Phenylephrine also lacks demonstrated effectiveness, and there are no studies of its safety in children. AAP clinical policy statements dating from 1997 have found no studies to support the safety or efficacy of dextromethorphan in pediatrics and no indications for its use. In small children, cough is an important protective mechanism to clear narrow airways, making suppression dangerous. Acetaminophen is added to pediatric cough and cold syrups for reduction of fever and pain. Overdoses are common and potentially toxic.

In children, dosing of drugs is uncertain, often approximated from adult studies. Potential interactions with other drugs or dietary supplements is a concern. According to the 2007 National Health Interview Survey, an estimated 2.9 million children and adolescents use some type of dietary supplement, yet many families fail to disclose supplement use to their child's clinician for fear of a negative response.

Each of these factors is important to consider in thinking about OTC drug use in children. Serious adverse effects and accidental overdose have been reported for every medicine Kim had in her system. The interaction of these drugs put Kim at great risk.

INTEGRATIVE MEDICINE APPROACHES TO TREATING UPPER RESPIRATORY ILLNESS IN CHILDREN

In non-urgent situations, an integrative approach to a common head cold can be quite effective. The following therapies have supporting evidence in pediatric URI:

- Nasal irrigation with saline; a humidifier in the child's bedroom
- Warm fluids by mouth to help thin mucus
- Buckwheat (dark) honey, in those over one year of age for reducing nighttime cough
- Vapor rub with menthol for congestion
- Oral zinc sulfate, in those over one year of age
- Umcka ColdCare, a homeopathic extract of a species of geranium *(Pelargonium sidoides),* which has some supporting evidence in children
- Elderberry syrup, which has been shown to be effective in fighting influenza and has a long history of use in children over one year of age

Conversely, therapies currently lacking supporting evidence in pediatric upper respiratory illness include antibiotics, OTC cough-cold medicines, echinacea, and vitamin C.

Acetaminophen or nonsteroidal anti-inflammatories (NSAIDs) may have a place in treatment if used judiciously for fever and pain; however, each carries its own risks (discussed in chapter 8). Accurate dosing of these medications is very important, especially in young children and infants.

Preventive precautions include standard immunizations, annual flu shots (if there are no existing contra-indications), regular hand washing with soap and water, and avoidance of crowds or school if the child is sick to allow time for rest and healing. Emerging research suggests some benefit of probiotics in prevention of acute URI in children. Trials involved a range of probiotic strains given over three months or longer. Use of oral zinc in liquid or lozenge form is associated with fewer colds in children.

The bottom line is that although clinicians often feel pressured by parents to write a prescription or recommend over-the-counter medicine for URIs, taking the time to discuss non-pharmaceutical options is at least as important and likely to be much safer for the child. In Kim's case, it is very possible that the emergency room visit with its associated stress and expense could have been avoided entirely if non-pharmaceutical approaches had been used from the start to relieve the symptoms of her head cold.

Luis

Luis is a thirteen-year-old boy with a diagnosis of metabolic syndrome (insulin resistance, elevated blood glucose, high blood pressure, abdominal obesity, abnormal blood fats). He arrived in the pediatric emergency department after fainting in physical education class during the first lap of a one-mile run. Students had seen

Luis drinking a canned energy drink just before the start of class. On arrival in the emergency department, he was alert but jittery and frightened. Cardiac workup quickly ruled out a serious heart problem. Vital signs showed a rapid heart rate and slightly elevated blood pressure. On questioning he admitted to drinking two 16-ounce energy drinks to help him get a good time on the run.

Luis was unaware that most energy drinks contain on average 70 to 240 milligrams of caffeine and 54 to 62 grams of sugar (13 to 15 teaspoons) per can. In comparison, a typical 12-ounce soda contains 35 milligrams of caffeine and 40 grams of sugar (10 teaspoons). Luis's fainting spell on overexertion, along with jitteriness and hypertension, are classic symptoms seen when energy drinks are taken in excess. Energy drinks and energy shots, heavily marketed to adolescents and young adults, accounted for $6.9 billion in sales in the United States in 2012. A 2011 AAP statement cautioned that children and adolescents should not consume energy drinks because of their high content of caffeine and sugar. Reports of adverse cardiovascular events, sleep and behavioral disorders, hypertension, seizures, and death have been recorded with their use, especially when they are combined with alcohol, a practice common in young adults.

A review of Luis's medical history showed that he

had experienced rapid weight gain since age nine. He had previously tried an over-the-counter version of orlistat (Alli), a drug used to treat obesity by blocking intestinal absorption of fats, but discontinued it due to uncomfortable side effects (flatulence and diarrhea). The parents stated that Luis's pediatrician had recently given him three prescriptions: one to lower blood sugar, a second to reduce cholesterol, and a third for depression, and had considered adding a fourth drug for blood pressure control. The parents filled the prescriptions but were alarmed at the list of potential side effects and wanted to help get Luis off the drugs.

A review of Luis's lifestyle habits showed frequent intake of processed foods high in sugar and flour, processed meats, sugary beverages, and energy drinks to "help him study" and "give him energy." He spent an average of six hours a day on video games, got only about seven hours of sleep a night, and rarely went outdoors. He took no regular exercise outside of school physical education twice a week. Luis acknowledged feeling depressed due to bullying but denied wanting to harm himself or others.

Overmedicating Obese Children

• Approximately one in three children in North America is overweight or obese, including those in preschool and elementary school.

• Obesity in childhood commonly persists into adulthood.

• The majority of obese children have at least one related medical condition, such as high blood pressure, that may require medication.

• Mental health issues such as anxiety, depression, social withdrawal, bullying, binge eating disorder, and low self-esteem are very common in obese children and are often treated with prescription medications.

• Insufficient sleep has been linked to overweight and obesity in children and may be treated with prescription or OTC medications. (Sleep aids are discussed in chapter 6.)

The medications prescribed for Luis are recommended routinely in cases of pediatric obesity:

Metformin

Used to treat insulin resistance, which often accompanies obesity, metformin (Glumetza, Glucophage) is also used "off label" to enhance weight loss in some obese children. (Its approved use in diabetes treatment is discussed in chapter 14.) Its most common side effects are nausea, vomiting, diarrhea, and increased gas. In adults, long-term treatment with metformin has been shown to increase the risk of vitamin B_{12} deficiency; long-term studies in children and adolescents are lacking.

Statins

Universal cholesterol screening is recommended between ages nine and eleven years to identify children at risk for abnormally high levels. We have very limited data on the impact of statins in children. (See chapter 2 for detailed information on these drugs.)

Antidepressants

Weight gain is a relatively common side effect of anti-depressant medications, a compounding problem for overweight adolescents like Luis. (Use of these and other psychiatric medications in children is discussed in chapter 10.)

Antihypertensives

Obese kids often have high blood pressure and are prescribed the same antihypertensive drugs used in adults. (These are discussed in detail in chapter 13.)

Orlistat

Sold over-the-counter as Alli and by prescription as Xenical, orlistat is a lipase inhibitor, meaning it inhibits the enzyme needed for breakdown of fats and prevents their absorption from foods. The main side effects are flatulence, oily loose stools, and oily spotting on clothes, which not surprisingly result in poor compliance.

Because it interferes with absorption of fat-soluble vitamins, orlistat can also affect growth and development. Long-term studies on its effects in children and adolescents are lacking.

Pediatric obesity is a prevalent and complex problem that resists pharmaceutical treatment. This has fueled interest in more extreme approaches, such as bariatric surgery in adolescents (gastric banding or bypass). Although surgery can result in weight loss and reversal of type 2 diabetes, it is associated with vitamin deficiencies, chronic malabsorption, and other significant risks and should be reserved for carefully screened, dangerously obese adolescents.

Integrative Medicine Approaches to Treating Obesity in Children

Expert consensus is that non-pharmacological approaches should be first-line treatments for obesity, yet few pediatricians are trained to help patients with comprehensive lifestyle change. This gap in medical education presents an important opportunity for integrative medicine practitioners, who are trained in these areas:

• Nutrition counseling to promote healthy whole foods in place of processed foods and sugary beverages

- Motivational interviewing to catalyze and support behavior change
- Mind-body therapies to manage anxiety and depression and cultivate self-regulation of emotions
- Advising about low-impact physical activities, such as yoga and tai chi
- Counseling on sleep hygiene
- Environmental health education to reduce exposures to endocrine-disrupting chemicals linked to obesity
- Use of selected dietary supplements to fill gaps in the diet, such as omega-3 fatty acids, vitamin D, and probiotics
- Promotion of family and community support to build positive social connections.

After the emergency department scare, Luis was determined to lose weight and stop all the medications. His pediatrician brought in a registered dietician and a behavioral therapist to help. Motivational interviewing enabled Luis to make the shift to a healthier diet and find physical activities he enjoyed. He eliminated the energy drinks. He tried clinical hypnosis and guided imagery along with breathing exercises to boost his self-esteem and cope with school challenges. Luis lost weight gradually and was able to wean off the medications over the course of a year. The following year he won a regional science fair prize for a project on their harmful effects.

BOTTOM LINE

Between them, Kim and Luis were put on a total of eight medications for the treatment of two common medical conditions. These included guaifenesin, dextromethorphan, phenylephrine, acetaminophen, amoxicillin, metformin, a statin, and an SSRI, each with potentially serious adverse effects. The caffeine in Luis's energy drinks added a potent stimulant to the tally. Kim's story highlights the risks involved with seemingly safe and easily available OTC medications. Luis's story emphasizes the dangers of direct marketing of stimulating beverages to children and the futility of relying on pharmaceutical treatment for lifestyle-driven diseases. Both parents and physicians should be alarmed at the widespread overuse of medications—in millions of children—for treatment of other common conditions such as asthma, attention deficit hyperactivity disorder (ADHD), autism, diabetes, arthritis, gastrointestinal disorders, anxiety, and depression.

The prevalence of medication use in children, along with the unpredictability of individual response and high risk of overdose, add up to a powerful argument for the role of integrative medicine in young patients. The emphasis should be on prevention, maximum engagement of the child's innate healing response, reduction of medications, and lifestyle counseling. I would argue that these approaches must be supported by proactive health care reform and fair insurance reimbursement.

17

Overmedication of the Elderly

After seventy-nine years of dealing with Wisconsin winters, Norman finally met his match in an unusually long and cold one. In the midst of what seemed like interminable snow, he surveyed the icy sidewalks and decided it was probably a good idea for him to discontinue his daily walks around the neighborhood and stay home.

With less physical activity, Norman found it frustratingly difficult to get to sleep. His wife suggested that he try over-the-counter (OTC) diphenhydramine (Benadryl). It seemed to work — he slept for a full eight hours the first time he used it. Norman continued to take the drug nightly, even after the snow and ice melted and he resumed his walks.

In the spring, Norman saw his primary care

physician for increasing difficulty urinating. The doctor prescribed terazosin (Hytrin), a medication that can help relieve urinary obstruction due to an enlarged prostate. His symptoms improved a bit.

Two months later, on standing up from a park bench on a warm summer's evening, Norman became light-headed and fell, fracturing his hip. After orthopedic surgery, he was given morphine to help manage his pain. To prevent the potentially serious constipation that is often a side effect of opioid drugs, his surgical team started him on Senna-S, a combination stool softener (docusate) and stimulant laxative (senna). His prior medications—diphenhydramine and terazosin—were continued as soon as he was able to swallow pills.

In the ensuing nights in the hospital, Norman became confused and combative and kept trying to get out of bed. To help calm him, the on-call team added lorazepam (Ativan), a benzodiazepine, to the mix of diphenhydramine, terazosin, docusate/senna, and morphine. After his hip fracture had healed enough for him to leave the hospital, Norman was discharged to a rehabilitation facility, still on all the medications.

Within a few days of his transfer, Norman developed redness and warmth at the site of the surgical incision. Suspecting a bacterial infection, the rehab physician gave him a course of an antibiotic, amoxicillin-clavulanate (Augmentin). A few days after starting this, Norman developed diarrhea. The attending physician stopped the Senna-S and started imodium (Loper-amide), a drug that slows intestinal movement.

The diarrhea soon resolved, but the stool softener/laxative was not resumed and the imodium continued. A week later, Norman complained of severe abdominal pain and was found to be totally constipated with concerning distension of the bowels ("toxic megacolon"). He was readmitted to the hospital, where he underwent emergency abdominal surgery. Because he could not take oral medicines, he was switched to intravenous morphine and lorazepam, with the addition of IV omeprazole (Prilosec—a proton pump inhibitor, or PPI) to decrease the acid in his stomach and minimize the risk of an ulcer developing. Once his GI tract healed, his diphenhydramine, terazosin, morphine, lorazepam, stool softener/laxative, and omeprazole were all resumed in oral formulations.

When he was deemed stable enough to leave the hospital, Norman was transferred to a skilled nursing facility. (He did not qualify for return to the rehab facility because he was not physically able to participate in the required four hours of physical therapy a day.) His medication list from the hospital went along with him. During his stay in this facility, Norman continued to have pain in his hip and leg, and because he seemed less vibrant and more subdued, the rehab doctor started him on amitriptyline (Elavil), an antidepressant that is also frequently used to help diminish pain. Eventually, Norman was sent home. His wife filled his home-going prescriptions for terazosin, morphine, lorazepam, amitriptyline, and omeprazole. And a bottle of over-the-counter diphenhydramine was dutifully waiting for him on his nightstand.

The following year, Norman's wife urged him to speak with his primary care physician about new memory problems and an increased tendency to fall. That doctor did document some memory impairment and also noted that Norman was unsteady on his feet, especially just after rising from a seated position. Blood pressure readings both seated and standing confirmed that he was experiencing orthostatic hypotension—a significant drop in blood pressure on standing up that can cause fainting and falling, a potential catastrophe for an older person with brittle bones. The physician explained the side effects associated with each of Norman's medications, and together they decided to stop all of them: diphenhydramine, terazosin, morphine, lorazepam, omeprazole, and amitriptyline. A few months later, Norman was able to walk outdoors with confidence, albeit with a little limp.

Stories like this are all too common among older adults. What started with a simple attempt to improve sleep with an over-the-counter remedy grew into a frightening scenario of overmedication with significant complications and adverse effects. In such cases, the involvement of different prescribers and caretakers, who have little direct communication with one another, often leads to the accumulation of more and more medications to help alleviate symptoms resulting from prior ones. And doctors are unlikely to stop medications prescribed by their peers.

OVERMEDICATING THE ELDERLY

As we age, we have more complaints and symptoms that seem made-to-order for pharmaceutical treatment. Medications like diphenhydramine and combinations of diphenhydramine and acetaminophen (such as Tylenol PM) are designed (or at least marketed) to help us fall asleep faster and stay asleep longer. These OTC remedies are particularly attractive to older people, many of whom find good sleep elusive. Unfortunately, although the sedating antihistamines can be effective, they do not provide the restorative natural sleep that the body and mind need. And they are fraught with potential side effects, which can be particularly dangerous in older people: worsening of urinary obstruction, increased risk of falling, greater likelihood of experiencing delirium, and a greater chance of being diagnosed with dementia*—all conditions that often prompt the administration

---

* Delirium is a temporary state of confusion, usually caused by fever, intoxication, medications, pain, or trauma. Dementia is progressive loss

of even more medications, each with its own potential for adverse effects on aging bodies and minds.

Whether Norman would have developed urinary obstruction if he had not taken the diphenhydramine cannot be determined. It is entirely plausible that his primary care physician was not aware that he was taking OTC diphenhydramine nightly. No one thought to try stopping the sleep aid to see if it was causing his urinary problem.

Terazosin is one of the most common drugs used to treat urinary retention. Although it helps to some extent, it also has an effect on blood vessels that can lead to orthostatic hypotension.

Upon admission to a hospital, there is a tendency among physicians to take the patient's medication list from home and add new meds to it. Norman's diphenhydramine and terazosin were continued for sleep and for urinary obstruction, with an opioid added to alleviate pain from the hip fracture. While opioids can be essential for control of severe pain, they have their own attendant side effects to be wary of, such as serious constipation. They can also increase the risk of falling and worsen urinary obstruction.

Studies of older hip fracture patients have shown that 16 to 62 percent develop delirium. Pain appears to

---

of memory and other mental abilities, often associated with Alzheimer's disease or diminished blood flow to the brain.

be a leading risk factor associated with delirium in this population. Possibly, Norman was not given enough morphine to control his pain (including the significant discomfort caused by a distended bladder and a blocked colon), but it is noteworthy that diphenhydramine on its own can cause delirium in older patients.

Although lorazepam can quickly quell agitation and make a combative patient docile, it is rarely the ideal solution because it does not address the underlying causes of the behavioral change. Moreover, benzodiazepines also increase the risk of falls and can even precipitate delirium by making people groggy and confused. The American Geriatrics Society felt so strongly about avoiding benzodiazepine use in the elderly that it included benzodiazepine prescribing in the "Five Things That Physicians and Patients Should Question" list for the geriatrics section of the Choosing Wisely educational campaign to improve doctor-patient relationships.

As commonly occurs in hospitalized patients today, Norman developed an infection, for which he was given a strong antibiotic. Antibiotic treatment kills not only the offending bacteria, but also the good bacteria in the intestines. Diarrhea is a frequent outcome of this drastic alteration in the normal gut flora. Hospitalized patients on antibiotics are also at risk for serious gut infection with *Clostridium difficile (C. diff)*. In Norman's case, forgetting to discontinue imodium and restart the bowel stimulant while he was still taking morphine probably led to paralysis of the gut and his toxic megacolon. Then, with his bowels not moving, his hospital team opted to put him on omeprazole to suppress acid production in his stomach. This drug can help prevent or treat a serious bleeding ulcer, but acidity in the stomach serves vital functions, and long-term suppression of it with drugs like omeprazole can have serious consequences (see chapter 3), including increased risk of *C. diff* infection.

The popularity of amitriptyline and related older (tricyclic) antidepressants has waned in psychiatry, but they are still used for the relief of chronic pain, even though their efficacy for this is questionable. Unfortunately for Norman, tricyclic antidepressants, like their antihistamine relatives, can cause urinary obstruction and constipation as well as increase the risk of falls and delirium.

Norman went from home to the hospital, from the hospital to rehab, then back to the hospital, and then to the skilled nursing facility before finally going home. With each change of venue and clinicians, the potential for medication errors increased.

INTEGRATIVE MEDICINE APPROACHES

As you can see from the chapters in this book, there are many ways to manage common complaints other than relying on medications. If Norman had found an indoor exercise routine to take the place of his walks around the neighborhood when the sidewalks were icy, his sleep might not have suffered. An integrative medicine practitioner could have advised him about sleep hygiene and suggested trying valerian or melatonin as natural sleep aids (see chapter 6).

If his primary care physician had asked Norman about any new OTC medicines he was taking, and advised that he try alternatives to diphenhydramine before prescribing terazosin for urinary retention, perhaps the fall and subsequent outcomes might have been different.

After the hip injury, appropriate pain relief and attention to urinary retention and constipation might have averted the episodes of delirium and obviated the need for lorazepam, which, especially in combination with opioids, can dangerously compromise breathing and impact cognitive function.

Had Norman been able to get good nightly sleep, he might have been able to tolerate his pain with less need for medication, and the risk of delirium might have been lower. But prolonged stays in a hospital or rehab facility or nursing home can cause a good night's sleep to be merely a distant memory and unfulfilled yearning. (See chapters 12 and 6 for suggestions about the non-pharmacological management of pain and insomnia.)

BOTTOM LINE

Too many older people are on too many medications, putting them at risk for serious adverse reactions and drug interactions. When I see the medicines that elderly patients and friends are taking, more often than not I note many drugs prescribed by different physicians, as well as a generous sampling of OTC medications. I wonder if anyone is overseeing all of it. Research suggests that in many instances the answer is no. Among those over the age of sixty-five, the incidence of polypharmacy, defined as being on five or more medications at one time, rose from 30.6 percent to 35.8 percent from 2005 to 2011, putting an estimated 15 percent of older adults at risk for complications from drug interactions. Further complicating matters, nearly two-thirds of older adults also take dietary supplements. Another third regularly uses OTC medication.

Older people grew up in era when medical doctors were more authoritarian and paternalistic; they are used to complying with doctors' orders and not questioning the need for medications. They may be more reluctant to ask a physician about an OTC product or dietary supplement. If Norman had felt that it was important and permissible to discuss his diphenhydramine use with his primary care physician, perhaps the cascade of untoward events that engulfed him would have been avoided.

If you have an elderly relative or friend on multiple medications, urge that person to consult a pharmacist for a medication therapy management (MTM) review (see chapter 18 for a description of this service).

As a patient or patient's advocate, you are responsible for keeping an updated list of what medications are prescribed, including the dosage, as well as the dates they were started or stopped or the dosage changed. Be sure to write down the reason for starting or stopping each medication or changing dosage.

It is critically important for each prescriber/caretaker to be thoroughly versed in a patient's medication history (including OTC products and herbal remedies, as well as use of alcohol and caffeine) and to communicate with *all* other caretakers and prescribers. Communication must be bidirectional, with open and nonjudgmental discussions encouraged among all concerned parties.

When an elderly patient enters a hospital, rehab, or chronic care facility, the caretaker must be able to advocate for him or her in those settings. It is much easier for an institution to administer a medication than it is to adjust the assault of continuous light and noise that may be disturbing sleep or causing agitation. But firm and reasoned insistence can persuade staff to make modifications. Speak directly with the nurse on duty as well as with the head nurse and the physician or prescriber. Explain your concerns and offer viable suggestions for alternatives. The common paramount goal of everyone should be the health and welfare of the patient.

To learn about safe and effective ways to manage chronic conditions and symptoms, including lifestyle change, natural remedies, and unconventional therapies, consult a health professional trained in integrative medicine.

Over-Reliance on Medications: A Pharmacist's View

By Kim DeRhodes, RPh

Wendy, age sixty-eight, made an appointment at an integrative medicine clinic because she wanted someone to look carefully at her medications; she felt she was taking too many. She was diabetic and had been diagnosed with early Alzheimer's disease about five years before. She lived alone and had been self-reliant for a long time, but she now feared the loss of her independence. Her main complaints were confusion, headache, jaw pain, and nausea, which occurred almost every day and had a significant negative impact on her life. She had difficulty sleeping and was drowsy during the daytime. Having lost thirty pounds over the past year, which she attributed to changes in her diet and level of activity, her diabetes was well controlled. She had seen three different doctors for her various health issues, who had put her on thirteen different prescription medications daily. In addition, she was taking several over-the-counter (OTC) medications and supplements. The integrative medicine physician referred her to a pharmacist for a medication therapy management (MTM) review, a service pharmacists are trained to provide.

What can you do to ensure that all the medications prescribed for you are appropriate? First, you should not assume that your medication list is being carefully reviewed at each doctor visit. Almost certainly, it is not. Even though your doctor may ask about all your medications, usually that is done just to meet the requirement of keeping an accurate and complete medication list in your medical record. An accurate medication list is not the same as an optimal medication list—especially if you are seeing more than one doctor. Doctors are hesitant to change medications prescribed by colleagues, even when they think a particular one is not right for a patient. Here is where pharmacists can help. They are truly the drug experts, yet they are an underused resource. Pharmacists have at least six years of professional training that equips them to do much more than just fill prescriptions. They serve in both hospitals and outpatient settings, dosing and managing drug therapy, counseling patients, and working with physicians and other health care professionals to provide drug information and optimize therapy. And their advice is often free.

It is important for every patient who is on five or more drugs to have an MTM session with a pharmacist, because the risk of an adverse drug reaction or drug interaction goes up exponentially when more than that number are prescribed. It is imperative for patients over the age of sixty-five to have this done. MTM can be thought of as a "medication checkup." Pharmacists provide the service to help patients get the most benefit from their prescription and OTC medications. They actively manage drug therapy by identifying and preventing medication-related problems as well as working with physicians to resolve them. People who may benefit the most include those who use several medications, have several health conditions, have questions about or problems with their medications, have been recently hospitalized, or obtain their medications from more than one pharmacy or physician.

MTM works best as a partnership among patients, pharmacists, physicians, and other caregivers to ensure safe, effective use of medications and achieve the desired outcomes from therapy. A well-trained pharmacist can also identify possible problems or interactions with vitamins, other dietary supplements, and herbal and other natural remedies. (One caution: At present, colleges of pharmacy do not provide adequate education about these products, covering them in just a few lectures or brief elective courses. All pharmacists have access to online information about interactions between drugs and supplements. They may not, however, be knowledgeable about the benefits of supplements.)

If you are on an expensive medicine, a pharmacist can often recommend a lower-cost alternative. It is not at all unusual for patients who are on multiple medications to save hundreds of dollars per year in prescription costs after optimizing their medication regimen. Here are some important questions to ask your pharmacist:

- Why am I on this medication?
- When and how should I take it?
- How long should I take it for?
- What are the side effects?
- Is there a less expensive alternative that would work just as well?
- Are there medication or supplement interactions I should be aware of?
- Does this medicine interact with alcohol or certain foods?
- Does this drug cause any nutrient deficiencies?
- Is there a medication I might benefit from that I am not taking for my condition?

Let's return to Wendy's situation. Remember that her main complaints were memory issues, headaches, nausea, jaw pain, difficulty sleeping, and daytime drowsiness. After the pharmacist reviewed her medication list, the following problems were identified:

• There is a well-documented drug interaction between two of the drugs she was taking, leading to adverse reactions including nausea and confusion.

• One of the drugs she was using is on the Beers List, a compilation of medications that are considered inappropriate for those over the age of sixty-five. The side effects of this particular drug include excessive central nervous system stimulation, sleep disturbances, and nausea. It is also associated with bruxism (teeth grinding at night), aching jaw, and headache, as well as severe memory loss.

• She was on a sleeping pill at night (also on the Beers List as inappropriate for someone her age) and a medication to increase alertness during the day with known side effects of headache, nausea, and dizziness. This is a glaring example of polypharmacy at its worst.

• She was on two different drugs for stomach acid. Long-term use of acid-suppressive drugs can cause deficiencies of vitamin B_{12} and magnesium; B_{12} deficiency is associated with cognitive problems.

• Memory loss and cognitive problems are also associated with the drug she was taking for high cholesterol.

When Wendy's physician made the changes the pharmacist recommended, Wendy regained normal cognitive function and most of her daily complaints disappeared.

Pharmacists are often able to spend thirty to sixty minutes with a patient, reviewing every aspect of drug therapy and uncovering hidden problems. They can help patients understand why they are on certain medications, whether there are less expensive but just as effective alternatives, whether a drug needs to be added to the treatment regimen, and whether a medication is no longer needed.

So, how do you go about having a medication therapy management session? Ask at the pharmacy where you get your prescriptions filled if one of the pharmacists there can provide one. If not, try asking the pharmacist at a local independently owned pharmacy (as opposed to a chain store); some even specialize in this service. MTM is usually provided for a nominal fee and can be free for Medicare patients. The money it can save will usually offset any cost involved.

You may ask, "Why can't doctors perform this service?" The sad fact is they just don't have the time. They also do not have as much in-depth knowledge of drugs, mostly relying on information from manufacturers rather than from objective sources. Your pharmacist will not make any drug therapy decision without first discussing it with your doctor. Your doctor is ultimately responsible for making any needed changes in your drug therapy, as pharmacists cannot prescribe medications unless they are working directly under the supervision of a physician.

In integrative medicine, we strive to use the best of all available therapies, both conventional and unconventional. In many cases, a prescription drug may well be the "best medicine." In other cases, the best medicine may be something else. Natural alternatives to drug therapy and treatments that do not involve drugs at all are often effective and less expensive. Don't expect a pill to cure everything that ails you. Take advantage of the little-known but extremely useful service: a medication therapy management session with a pharmacist. It could improve your health, save you money, and spare you the pain and suffering of drug interactions and side effects.

Last Words

It is in the interest of all of us — patients, doctors, nurses, pharmacists, other health care professionals, parents, and our elected representatives — to reduce overmedication in our society. I have told you as clearly as I can why our excessive reliance on medication is a problem. We all have work to do if we want to resolve it.

If you are a consumer, be informed. Do not take medications, whether prescribed or available over the counter or sold online or in health food stores, unless you know the reason for taking them, understand how they work, and can weigh potential benefits against potential risks. Also, I urge you to find out whether safe and effective nondrug methods are available to manage any health conditions you have. If you decide that medication therapy is indicated, try to use less potent drugs rather than more potent ones, starting with the lowest dosage that works for you. This may be easier if you make appropriate lifestyle changes and experiment with natural remedies and other therapies, which may also enable you to shorten the duration of medication treatment. Pay attention to side effects, be wary of adverse drug reactions and interactions, and if you are on multiple medications, consult a pharmacist for a medication therapy management session.

Keep in mind that doctors are frequently paid thousands of dollars to promote drugs to other doctors and allied health care professionals. The cozy (and lucrative) relationship between the pharmaceutical industry and physicians has become such a problem that the Affordable Care Act mandates public disclosure of these payments. There is now a website you can check to see if your doctor has taken money from the pharmaceutical industry: cms.gov/openpayments.

If you are a pharmacist, please become knowledgeable about the dietary supplements, herbal remedies, and other natural products that so many consumers are taking. Be able to give advice about their safety, efficacy, and possible side effects and interactions with prescribed and over-the-counter (OTC) drugs. Through your professional organizations, try to influence colleges of pharmacy to include these topics in their curriculums. Also let consumers know about the services you offer to help them use medications wisely.

If you are a physician, nurse, or allied health care provider, I have a number of suggestions:

• Seek out nonbiased information on medications you prescribe or recommend, rather than relying on product information supplied by manufacturers.

• Insist that patients disclose all the products they are taking: prescribed and OTC drugs, dietary supplements, herbal remedies, and so on. If you are not sure about possible adverse reactions and drug interactions, consult a knowledgeable pharmacist.

• Get a sense of the lifestyle habits of your patients. Take dietary histories from them. Know what lifestyle modifications may be used as primary interventions for common health conditions, and become familiar with motivational interviewing as a technique to encourage patients to change habits.

• Be informed about alternatives to medication therapy for the health conditions you see most often. Know how to make appropriate referrals to other practitioners: registered dietitians, for example, or mind-body therapists.

• Learn about integrative medicine approaches for managing common health conditions.

If you are a parent, protect your children from over-medication by knowing the facts about any prescribed or OTC drugs you give them. Avoid using antibiotics unless they are absolutely necessary. The good news is that growing numbers of pediatricians are trained in integrative medicine; they can help you manage common health conditions in children with less emphasis on medication.

I don't know what I can suggest to curb the worst practices of the pharmaceutical industry, except to express my hope that all readers of this book will contact their elected representatives to demand an end to direct-to-consumer advertising of prescription medications.

For some years now, I have called for the US Food and Drug Administration to create a new division of Natural Therapeutic Agents to regulate dietary supplements, herbal remedies, and other natural products marketed for health benefits. Its purpose would be to ensure that products of this sort are safe and effective, not to thwart consumer access to them. Labeling should give indications for use as well as recommended dosage. Other countries—Canada and Germany, for instance—do a better job of this than the United States does.

Colleges of medicine, nursing, and pharmacy must provide adequate education about natural therapeutic agents.

I firmly believe that integrative medicine is the way of the future. It uses medication therapy as one way to manage disease and improve health, only when necessary and always in the context of a comprehensive treatment plan that addresses lifestyle issues and also makes use of nondrug therapies. One day, I am sure, we will be able to drop the word "integrative." This will simply be good medicine.

Acknowledgments

In March 2015 my friend and colleague Victoria Maizes, MD, executive director of the University of Arizona Center for Integrative Medicine, convened a think tank of graduates and faculty of the Center to plan the future course of the field and identify ways that we might influence the future of health care. Early in our discussions we agreed that overmedication in our society is a top priority and that integrative medicine can help reduce it. I first thought of a book on the subject during the meeting, and I thank Victoria for inspiring me to write it.

My agent, Richard Pine of InkWell Management, strongly encouraged me to work on it, as did my editor, Tracy Behar, of Little, Brown. I am most grateful for their support and efforts to get the manuscript ready for publication.

I could not have completed the book without the help of another friend and colleague, Russell Greenfield, MD, who not only edited chapter drafts and compiled references but also kept the contributors to their deadlines and supplied information for the chapter on cold and flu medications. Big thanks to him.

I also thank the contributors listed on pages ix to xiv. The research they did for me was invaluable. And I thank all the patients who let me use their stories about experiences with medications.

My assistant, Nancy Olmstead, kept my office in order. She and my business partner, Richard Baxter, managed my schedule so that I had time to write.

Finally, I thank my canine companions, Ajax and Juno, who were a constant presence by my desk throughout my work on the book.

Tucson, Arizona
June 2016

Resources

Practitioners of Integrative Medicine

The University of Arizona Center for Integrative Medicine has graduated 1,500 physicians as well as nurse practitioners and physician's assistants from intensive fellowship training in integrative medicine. You can look up graduates by specialty and location through the Center's website: azcim.org. Click on the "Find an Integrative Health Professional" link.

The American Board of Integrative Medicine (abpsus.org/integrative-medicine) provides board certification for qualified physicians trained in integrative medicine.

Integrative Medicine Treatments for Common Health Conditions

My website (DrWeil.com) has evidence-based information on a great many health conditions and integrative approaches to managing them.

See also my book *Natural Health, Natural Medicine: The Complete Guide to Wellness and Self-Care for Optimum Health* (Boston/New York, Houghton Mifflin, rev. ed., 2004).

I am the general editor of the Weil Integrative Medicine Library, a series of volumes for clinicians published by Oxford University Press: global.oup.com/academic/content/series/w/weil-integrative-medicine-library-iml. To date, the series includes volumes on Cardiology, Dermatology, Men's Health, Nursing, Oncology, Pain Management, Pediatrics, Psychiatry, Rheumatology, and Women's Health, with others in preparation. Each volume gives detailed, evidence-based information on the integrative medicine approach to treating health conditions dealt with by these specialties. Although these are academic books, anyone can use them as reference works. You can also direct your health care providers to them.

Another excellent resource for practitioners is the textbook *Integrative Medicine* by David Rakel, MD, 3rd ed. (Philadelphia: Elsevier, 2012).

National Institutes of Health (NIH)

The National Center for Complementary and Integrative Health (nccih.nih.gov) conducts research on complementary, alternative, and integrative treatments. The website has a great deal of information on health topics.

The Office of Dietary Supplements (ods.od.nih.gov) is a good source of information on vitamins, minerals, and other dietary supplements.

Safe Disposal of Medications

The best way to dispose of old and unwanted medications is to bring them to an approved location on one of the Drug Enforcement Administration's National Prescription Drug Take-Back Days. See deadiversion.usdoj.gov/drug_disposal/takeback for details.

Notes

Too Many Meds: The Problem — and the Solution

3: **About half of us are now taking at least one:** National Center for Health Statistics (NCHS). "Health, United States, 2013: With Special Feature on Prescription Drugs." Hyattsville, MD, 2014. http://www.cdc.gov/nchs/data/hus/hus13.pdf.

3: **Use of over-the-counter (OTC) medications has exploded just as dramatically:** American College of Preventive Medicine (ACPM). "Over-the-counter medications: use in general and special populations, therapeutic errors, misuse, storage and disposal." 2011. http://www.acpm.org/?OTCMeds_ClinRef.

3: **And more of us than ever are consuming dietary supplements, herbal remedies, and other products:** National Center for Health Statistics (NCHS). "Dietary supplement use among U.S. adults has increased since NHANES III (1998–2004)." Last updated April 13, 2011. http://www.cdc.gov/nchs/products/databriefs/db61.htm.

5: **Much evidence links the Mediterranean diet with good health, longevity, and low risk of disease:** Salas-Salvadó J, Guasch-Ferré M, Lee CH, et al. "Protective effects of the Mediterranean diet on type 2 diabetes and metabolic syndrome." *J Nutr* 2016;146:920S–927S.

5: **The DASH diet is an effective intervention for lowering high blood pressure:** Craddick SR, Elmer PJ, Obarzanek E, et al. "The DASH diet and blood pressure." *Curr Atheroscler Rep* 2003;5:484–91.

9: **Hundreds of thousands of deaths occur each year in the United States as a result of adverse drug reactions:** Lazarou J, Pomeranz BH, Corey PN. "Incidence of adverse drug reactions in hospitalized patients: a meta-analysis of prospective studies." *JAMA* 1998;279:1200–1205.

17: **Per-person spending on drugs in our country is close to $1,000 annually:** Organization for Economic Co-operation and Development (OECD). "Health at a Glance 2015. Pharmaceutical expenditure." http://www.keepeek.com/Digital-Asset-Management/oecd/social-issues-migration-health/health-at-a-glance-2015/pharmaceutical-expenditure_health_glance-2015-65-en#page1.

17: **US spending for prescription drugs is close to $300 billion per year:** Kessler G. "Trump's truly absurd claim he would save $300 billion a year on prescription drugs." *Washington Post,* February 18, 2016. https://www.washingtonpost.com/news/fact-checker/wp/2016/02/18/trumps-truly-absurd-claim-he-would-save-300-billion-a-year-on-prescription-drugs/.

Chapter 1. Antibiotics

23: **fecal microbial transplant (FMT), a cutting-edge treatment for digestive infections resistant to antibiotics:** Zanella Terrier MC, Simonet ML, Bichard P, et al. "Recurrent *Clostridium difficile* infections: the importance of the intestinal microbiota." *World J Gastroenterol* 2014;20:7416–23.

24: **Every year about 500,000 people in the United States acquire *C. diff* infections; about 30,000 people die as a result:** Centers for Disease Control and Prevention (CDC). "Healthcare-associated infections (HAIs)." Last updated September 23, 2015. http://www.cdc.gov/HAI/organisms/cdiff/Cdiff_clinicians.html.

25: **In 2009, Americans spent almost $11 billion on antibiotic therapy.** Suda KJ, Hicks LA, Roberts RM, et al. "A national evaluation of antibiotic expenditures by healthcare setting in the United States, 2009." *J Antimicrob Chemother* (2012) doi: 10.1093/jac/dks 445.

25: **Resistant infections now account for $20 billion in annual health care costs.** Tracy T, "White House proposes doubling spending on antibiotics." *Wall Street Journal,* January 27, 2015.

26: **livestock consumed a whopping 32 million pounds of antibiotics in 2012:** Food and Drug Administration (FDA). "2012 Summary report on antimicrobials sold or distributed for use in food-producing animals." September 2014. http://www.fda.gov/downloads/ForIndustry/User

Fees/AnimalDrugUserFeeActADUFA/UCM416983
.pdf.

27: **she reacted to it in much the same way as she had responded to the blueberry pie:** Graham F, Begin P, Paradis L, et al. "Streptomycin in a blueberry pie? Risk of allergic sensitization and reaction to antibiotics contained in foods." *J Allerg Clin Immunol* 2013;131:AB215.

28: **Those that had received the antibiotic reacted much more strongly to the spores:** Noverr MC, Noggle RM, Toews GB, et al. "Role of antibiotics and fungal microbiota in driving pulmonary allergic responses." *Infect Immunol* 2004;72:4996–5003.

28: **one of the important roles of normal gut flora is to resist colonization by pathogenic organisms:** Blaser M. "Antibiotic overuse: stop the killing of beneficial bacteria." *Nature* 2011;476:393–94.

28: **One study found that after a single treatment with intravenous antibiotics, fecal bacteria tests demonstrated a significant change in the variety of bacterial strains, as well as the presence and growth of *C. difficile:*** Ambrose NS, Johnson M, Burdon DW, et al. "The influence of single dose intravenous antibiotics on faecal flora and emergence of *Clostridium difficile.*" *J Antimicrob Chemother* 1985;15:319–26.

29: **Changes in the microbiome due to antibiotics have even been linked with obesity:** Gerard P. "Gut microbiota and obesity." *Cell Mol Life Sci* 2016;73:147–62.

31: **A review of thirty-one randomized studies found that when probiotic supplements are given along with anti-**

biotics, they reduce the risk of developing digestive symptoms: Goldenberg JZ, Ma SSY, Saxton JD, et al. "The use of probiotics to prevent *C. difficile* diarrhea associated with antibiotic use." *Cochrane Libr* 2013. doi: 10.1002/14651858.CD006095.pub3.

31: **And several studies show that spending sustained time in the forest boosts immune function:** Li Q. "Effect of forest bathing trips on human immune function." *Environ Health Prev Med* 2010;15:9–17.

31: **These protective phytonutrients enhance immunity:** Lee RJ, Cohen NA. "Role of bitter taste receptor T2R38 in upper respiratory infection and chronic rhinosinusitis." *Curr Opin Allergy Clin Immunol* 2015;15:14–20.

31: **Raw, unprocessed honey also can boost immunity:** Asama T, Arima T-H, Gomi T, et al. "*Lactobacillus kunkeei* YB38 from honeybee products enhances IgA production in healthy adults." *J Appl Microbiol* 2015; 119:818–26.

32: **Some botanicals can also boost immunity and help prevent infection:** Schapowal A, Klein P, Johnston SL. "Echinacea reduces the risk of recurrent respiratory tract infections and complications: a meta-analysis of randomized controlled trials." *Avd Ther* 2015;32:187–200. Cho WC, Leung KN. "In vitro and in vivo immunomodulating and immunorestorative effects of *Astragalus membranaceus.*" *J Ethnopharmacol* 2007;113:132–41.

32: **So can medicinal mushrooms:** Wachtel-Galor S, Yuen J, Buswell JA, et al. "Ganoderma lucidum (Lingzhi or Reishi): a medicinal mushroom." In: Benzie IFF,

Wachtel-Galor S, eds. *Herbal Medicine: Biomolecular and Clinical Aspects.* 2nd ed. (Boca Raton, FL: CRC Press/Taylor & Francis, 2011), chapter 9. Coy C, Standish LJ, Bender G, et al. "Significant correlation between TLR2 agonist activity and TNF-α induction in J774.A1 macrophage cells by different medicinal mushroom products." *Int J Med Mushrooms* 2015;17:713–22.

32: **Thyme and sage, as extracts or infusions in honey, also have antimicrobial properties:** Seibel J, Pergola C, Werz O, et al. "Bronchipret syrup containing thyme and ivy extracts suppresses bronchoalveolar inflammation and goblet cell hyperplasia in experimental bronchoalveolitis." *Phytomedicine* 2015;22:1172–77.

32: **Studies done on essential oils of eucalyptus, tea tree, lemongrass, and others:** Warnke PH, Lott AJ, Sherry E, et al. "The ongoing battle against multi-resistant strains: in-vitro inhibition of hospital-acquired MRSA, VRE, *Pseudomonas,* ESBL *E. coli* and *Klebsiella* species in the presence of plant-derived antiseptic oils." *J Craniomaxillofac Surg* 2013;41:321–26.

33: **Also learn to use natural products that are safe and effective treatments for minor infections, like tea tree oil *(Melaleuca alternifolia)* for skin and periodontal problems:** Pazyar N, Yaghoobi R, Bagherani N, et al. "A review of applications of tea tree oil in dermatology." *Int J Dermatol* 2013;52:784–90.

33: **and Oregon grape root *(Mahonia aquifolium)* for the gastrointestinal tract:** "Berberine." *Altern Med Rev* 2000;5:175–77.

Chapter 2. Statins

38: **a whopping 26 percent of adults in the United States are now taking a statin, at an annual cost to the health care system of more than $20 billion:** Gu Q P-RR, Burt VL, Kit, BK. "Prescription cholesterol-lowering medication use in adults aged 40 and over: United States, 2003–2012." Hyattsville, MD: National Center for Health Statistics, 2014.

38: **as many as half of all adult Americans are candidates for statin therapy:** Pencina MJ, Navar-Boggan AM, D'Agostino RB, Sr., et al. "Application of new cholesterol guidelines to a population-based sample." *N Engl J Med* 2014;370(15):1422–31.

38: **according to pediatric guidelines that now call for drug treatment in children as young as ten years old:** National Heart, Lung, and Blood Institute (NHLBI). "Expert panel on integrated guidelines for cardiovascular health and risk reduction in children and adolescents: Summary report." *Pediatrics* 2011;128(suppl 5):S213–56.

39: **In the best studies, statins reduce the chance of a heart attack in those at risk by no more than one-third:** Gutierrez J, Ramirez G, Rundek T, et al. "Statin therapy in the prevention of recurrent cardiovascular events: A sex-based meta-analysis." *Arch Intern Med* 2012;172(12): 909–19.

40: **In one recent study, 25 percent of individuals on statin therapy experienced it:** Cohen JD, Brinton EA, Ito MK, et al. "Understanding Statin Use in America and Gaps in Patient Education (USAGE): An Internet-based survey of 10,138 current and former statin users." *J Clin Lipidol* 2012;6(3):208–15.

40–41: **among patients who reported muscle symptoms, 47 percent of the time physicians immediately dismissed the possibility that the drug was to blame:** Golomb BA, McGraw JJ, Evans MA, et al. "Physician response to patient reports of adverse drug effects: implications for patient-targeted adverse effect surveillance." *Drug Saf* 2007;30(8):669–75.

42: **only one new case of statin-induced diabetes will occur among 250 patients after four years of treatment:** Shah RV, Goldfine AB. "Statins and risk of new-onset diabetes mellitus." *Circulation* 2012;126(18):e282–84.

43: **Although some CoQ10 studies have shown an improvement in statin side effects, most have not:** Banach M, Serban C, Sahebkar A, et al. "Effects of coenzyme Q10 on statin-induced myopathy: a meta-analysis of randomized controlled trials." *Mayo Clin Proc* 2015;90(1):24–34.

45: **Meditation is also remarkably beneficial:** Schneider RH, Grim CE, Rainforth MV, et al. "Stress reduction in the secondary prevention of cardiovascular disease: randomized, controlled trial of transcendental meditation and health education in Blacks." *Circ Cardiovasc Qual Outcomes* 2012;5(6):750–58.

45: **In a randomized trial, 85 percent of patients who could not tolerate prescription statins were able to take red yeast rice without side effects:** Becker DJ,

Gordon RY, Halbert SC, et al. "Red yeast rice for dyslipidemia in statin-intolerant patients: a randomized trial." *Ann Intern Med* 2009;150(12):830–39, W147–839.

Chapter 3. Medications for GERD

47–48: **except in very rare circumstances, overproduction of acid is not to blame:** Dunbar KB, Agaston T, et al. "Association of acute gastroesophageal reflux disease with esophageal histologic changes." *JAMA* 2016;315 (19):2104–12.

48: **About 113 million prescriptions for them are filled globally each year:** Perks, B. "Proton pump inhibitors are associated with increased risk of heart attack." *Pharmaceut J* June 16, 2015. http://www.pharmaceutical-journal.com/news-and-analysis/proton-pump-inhibitors-are-associated-with-increased-risk-of-heart-attack/20068748.article.

48: **Several years ago the total cost expenditure on PPIs was more than $13 billion:** Chubineh S, Birk J. "Proton pump inhibitors: the good, the bad, and the unwanted." *S Med J* 2012;105:613–18.

53: **upon cessation, most of them experienced acid-related symptoms:** Reimer C, Søndergaard B, Hilsted L, et al. "Proton-pump inhibitor therapy induces acid-related symptoms in healthy volunteers after withdrawal of therapy." *Gastroenterol* 2009;137:80–7, 87.e1.

53: **Long-term use of acid-suppressing drugs can inhibit normal, beneficial organisms, while encouraging overgrowth of harmful bacteria:** Imhann F, Bonder MJ,

Vich Vila A, et al: "Proton pump inhibitors affect the gut microbiome." *Gut* 2016;65:740–48.

54: **Some studies suggest there may be a higher rate of pneumonia in those taking H2s and PPIs:** Eom CS, Jeon CY, Lim JW, et al. "Use of acid-suppressive drugs and risk of pneumonia: a systematic review and meta-analysis." *CMAJ* 2011;183:310–9.

54: **Reduced gastric acidity can promote bacterial overgrowth in the small intestine:** Freedberg DE, Toussaint NC, Chen SP, et al. "Proton pump inhibitors alter specific taxa in the human gastrointestinal microbiome: a crossover trial." *Gastroenterol* 2015;149:883–85.e9

54: **PPI therapy can block calcium absorption, leading to osteoporosis and fractures:** Khalili H, Hunag ES, Jacobson BC, et al. "Use of proton pump inhibitors and risk of hip fracture in relation to dietary and lifestyle factors: a prospective cohort study." *BMJ* 2012;344 e372.

55: **A recent study brought to light the possibility of an increased risk of heart attack in patients using PPIs long term:** Shah NH, LePendu P, Bauer-Mehren A, et al. "Proton pump inhibitor usage and the risk of myocardial infarction in the general population." *PLoS One* 2015;10:e0124653.

55: **Evidence suggests an association between PPI use, kidney inflammation, and increased risk of chronic kidney disease:** Lazarus B, Chen Y, Wilson FP, et al. "Proton pump inhibitor use and the risk of chronic kidney disease." *JAMA Intern Med* 2016;285:2583–93.

55: **"The results emphasize the importance of limiting PPI use to only when it is medically necessary, and also limiting the duration of use to the shortest duration possible.":** Harrison P. "PPIs and kidney injury: longer use tied to higher risk." *Medscape* April 14, 2016. http://www.medscape.com/viewarticle/861991. Xie Y, Bowe B, Li T, et al. "Proton pump inhibitors and risk of incident CKD and progression to ESR." *J Am Soc Nephrol* 2016. Published online before print. doi: 10.1681/ASN. 2015121377.

55: **A study examining the use of PPIs in people age seventy-five and older showed that taking the medication was associated with a 44 percent increased risk of dementia:** Gomm W, von Holt K, Thome F, et al. "Association of proton pump inhibitors with risk of dementia: a pharmacoepidemiological claims data analysis." *JAMA Neurol* 2016;73:410–16.

57: **Following a gluten-free diet improves symptoms of GERD in those with celiac disease:** Nachman F, Vázquez H, Gonzalez A, et al. "Gastroesophageal reflux symptoms in patients with celiac disease and the effects of a gluten-free diet." *Clin Gastroenterol Hepatol* 2011;9:214–9.

57: **A recent study of GERD patients showed that feeling stressed was the most common lifestyle factor correlated with the disorder, present in 45.6 percent of 12,653 patients surveyed:** Haruma K, Kinoshita Y, Sakamoto S, et al. "Lifestyle factors and efficacy of lifestyle interventions in gastroesophageal reflux disease in patients with functional dyspepsia: primary care perspectives from the LEGEND study." *Intern Med* 2015;54:695–701.

59: **Ginger has been shown in numerous studies to help with nausea:** Wu K-L, Rayner CK, Chuah S-K, et al. "Effects of ginger on gastric emptying and motility in healthy humans." *Eur J Gastroenterol Hepatol* 2008;20: 436–40.

60: **one study showed it [melatonin] to be as effective as a PPI when used in combination with other supplements:** Pereira Rde S. "Regression of gastroesophageal reflux disease symptoms using dietary supplementation with melatonin, vitamins and amino acids: comparison with omeprazole." *J Pineal Res* 2006;41:195–200.

Chapter 4. Antihistamines

62: **an anti-inflammatory diet:** Weil A. *Healthy Aging* (New York: Alfred A. Knopf, 2005), chapter 9, 140–60. http://www.drweil.com/drw/u/ART02012/anti-inflammatory -diet.

65: **Among the most commonly sold OTC medications in the United States are cough-cold and allergy remedies, many of which are, or include, antihistamines:** Kaufman DW, Kelly JP, Rosenberg L, et al. "Recent patterns of medication use in the ambulatory adult population of the United States: the Slone Survey." *JAMA* 2002;287(3):337–44.

65: **In fact, they [these older antihistamines] can impair driving ability as much as or more than alcohol:** Weiler JM, Bloomfield JR, Woodworth GG, et al. "Effects of fexofenadine, diphenhydramine, and alcohol on driving performance: a randomized, placebo-controlled trial in the Iowa driving simulator." *Ann Intern Med* 2000;132(5):354–63.

66: **Taking such medications for the equivalent of three years or more increased the risk of developing dementia by 54 percent:** Gray SL, Anderson ML, Dublin S, et al. "Cumulative use of strong anticholinergics and incident dementia: a prospective cohort study." *JAMA Intern Med* 2015;175(3):401–407.

66–67: **several studies show that people who report regular long-term use of antihistamines are nearly three times as likely as non-users to develop these tumors:** Scheurer ME, Amirian ES, Davlin SL, et al. "Effects of antihistamine and anti-inflammatory medication use on risk of specific glioma histologies." *Int J Cancer* 2011;129:2290–96.

67: **an inverse relationship between allergies and glioma is one of the most consistent associations in the brain tumor literature:** McCarthy BJ, Rankin K, Il'yasova D, et al. "Assessment of type of allergy and antihistamine use in the development of glioma." *Cancer Epidemiol Biomarkers Prev* 2011;20(2);370–8.

67: **Drug therapy for allergies, taken as a whole and including OTC medications, costs more than $6 billion per year. An individual taking a second-generation**

antihistamine could spend anywhere from $8 to more than $200 per month. Goodman MJ, Jhaveri M, Saverno K, et al. "Cost-effectiveness of second-generation antihistamines and montekulast in relieving allergic rhinitis symptoms." *Am Health Drug Benefits* 2008:1:26–34. *Consumer Reports.* 2013. "Best buy drugs. Using the antihistamines to treat allergies, hay fever & hives: comparing effectiveness, safety, and price." http://consumer healthchoices.org/wp-content/uploads/2012/02/BBD -Antihistamines-Full.pdf.

68: **In a randomized, double-blind study of nearly one hundred patients, 57 percent rated nettle effective:** Mittman P. "Randomized, double-blind study of freeze-dried *Urtica dioica* in the treatment of allergic rhinitis." *Planta Med* 1990;56:44–7.

68: **A study of 132 people with hay fever found that an extract of this herb [butterbur] was as effective as cetirizine (Zyrtec) with fewer side effects:** Schapowal A, Petasites Study Group. "Randomised controlled trial of butterbur and cetirizine for treating seasonal allergic rhinitis." *BMJ* 2002;324(7330):144–6.

69: **emotions can powerfully mitigate the effects of allergen exposure:** Kimata H. "Effect of humor on allergen-induced wheal reactions." *JAMA* 2001;285(6):738.

Chapter 5. Medications for the Common Cold and the Flu

72: **Colds are also the most common acute human illness:** Heikkinen T, Järvinen A. "The common cold." *Lancet* 2003;361:51–9.

73: **colds are associated with an enormous economic burden:** Frendrick AM, Monto AS, Nightengale B, et al. "The economic burden of non-influenza-related viral respiratory tract infection in the United States." *Arch Intern Med* 2003;163:487–94.

73: **According to World Health Organization estimates, between three and five million cases of flu-related illness occur annually, as well as 250,000 to 500,000 flu-related deaths:** World Health Organization (WHO). "Influenza Fact Sheet." March 2014. http://www.who.int/mediacentre/factsheets/ fs211/en/.

73: **the flu leads to more than 400,000 hospitalizations and thousands of deaths each year, most involving the elderly:** Gasparini R, Amicizia D, Lai PL, et al. "Compounds with anti-influenza activity—present and future of strategies for optimal treatment and management of influenza. Part 1: Influenza life-cycle and currently available drugs." *J Prev Health Hyg* 2014;55:69–85.

74: **Most experts believe that vaccination provides some measure of protection:** Centers for Disease Control and Prevention (CDC). "Key facts about seasonal flu vaccine." Last updated October 2, 2015. http://www.cdc.gov/flu/protect/keyfacts.htm.

74: **Studies suggest that it can reduce the risk of heart attack:** Hebsur S, Vakil E, Oetgen WJ, et al. "Influenza and coronary artery disease: exploring a clinical association with myocardial infarction and analyzing the utility of vaccination in preventing myocardial infarction." *Rev Cardiovasc Med* 2014;15:168–75.

74–75: **reviews of data from healthy vaccinated individuals suggest a modest benefit at best and question the wisdom of widespread annual flu vaccination:** Demicheli V, Jefferson T, Al-Ansary LA, et al. "Vaccines for preventing influenza in healthy adults." *Cochrane Database Syst Rev* 2014;3:CD001269.

75: **A list of vaccines and their thimerosal content is available from the US Food and Drug Administration:** Food and Drug Administration (FDA). "Vaccine safety: thimerosal in vaccines." Last updated October 27, 2015. http://www.cdc .gov/vaccinesafety/concerns/thimerosal/.

75: **Nor do antibiotics have a role in preventing complications:** Kenealy T, Arroll B. "Antibiotics for the common cold and acute purulent rhinitis." *Cochrane Database Syst Rev* 2013;6:CD000247.

75: **In fact, a whopping 41 percent of all antibiotic prescriptions are directed against respiratory infections:** Shapiro DJ, Hicks LA, Pavia AT, et al. "Antibiotic prescribing for adults in ambulatory care in the USA, 2007– 2009." *J Antimicrob Chemother* 2014;69:234–40.

76: **Studies show that NAIs shorten the duration of flu by about one day only:** Jefferson T, Jones MA, Doshi P, et al. "Neuraminidase inhibitors for preventing and treating influenza in healthy adults and children." *Cochrane Database Syst Rev* 2014;10:4:CD008965. doi: 10.1002/14651858. Dobson J, Whitley RJ, Pocock S, et al. "Oseltamivir treatment for influenza in adults: a meta-analysis of randomized controlled trials." *Lancet* 2015;385:1729–37.

76: **And just as bacteria have become resistant to antibiotics, the flu virus is beginning to develop resistance to NAIs, specifically to oseltamivir:** Spanakis N, Pitiriga V, Gennimata, V, et al. "A review of neuraminidase inhibitor susceptibility in influenza strains." *Expert Rev Anti Infect Ther* 2014;12:1325–36. Nitsch-Osuch A, Brydak LB. "Influenza viruses resistant to neuraminidase inhibitors." *ACTA BP* 2014;61:505–8.

80–81: **Chronic stress, lack of social support, and depression can all interfere with immune function, increasing risk of infection:** Kiecolt-Glaser J, Cohen S, Janicki-Deverts D, et al. "Chronic stress, glucocorticoid receptor resistance, inflammation, and disease risk." *PNAS* 2012;109:5995–99.

81: **Mindfulness meditation has been shown to reduce the incidence, severity, and duration of cold symptoms, as has moderate exercise:** Barrett B, Hayney MS, Muller D, et al. "Meditation or exercise for preventing acute respiratory infection: a randomized controlled trial." *Ann Fam Med* 2012;10:337–46.

Chapter 6. Sleep Aids

83: **Women, the elderly, and highly educated people use more of them:** Chong Y, Fryar CD, Gu Q. "Prescription sleep aid use among adults: United States, 2005–2010." *NCHS data brief no. 127.* Hyattsville, MD: National Center for Health Statistics, 2013.

85: **40 million Americans have a chronic sleep disorder and 62 percent of American adults experience a sleep**

problem a few nights per week: Statistic Brain. "Sleeping disorder statistics." Research date April 12, 2015. http://www.statisticbrain.com/sleeping-disorder-statistics/.

85: **Poor sleep has been linked to chronic inflammation and increased risk for a broad range of illnesses:** Kryger MM, Roth T, Dement WC. *Principles and practice of sleep medicine.* 5th ed. (Philadelphia: Saunders, 2010).

85: **Medical conditions that cause pain or discomfort, or disrupt energy, as well as many commonly used medications, can also predispose us to, precipitate, or perpetuate insomnia:** Kryger, Roth, Dement, *Principles and practice of sleep medicine.*

86: **the National Sleep Foundation, the leading nonprofit organization dedicated to improving sleep health, has received substantial funds from numerous pharmaceutical companies:** Griffith D, Wiegand S. "A little too cozy? Not-for-profits may have undisclosed funding ties to for-profit companies." *Sacramento Bee.* July 13, 2005. http://www.pharmadisclose.org/spgppd/sb050713.html.

87: **More specifically, they [BDZs] increase light sleep at the expense of deep sleep, and they suppress dream sleep (REM):** Saddichha S. "Diagnosis and treatment of chronic insomnia." *Ann Indian Acad Neurol* 2010;13:94–102.

88: **Z-drugs should not be combined with alcohol or other sedating medications:** Huedo-Medina TB, Kirsch I, Middlemass, J, et al. "Effectiveness of nonbenzodiazepine hypnotics in treatment of adult insomnia: meta-analysis of data submitted to the FDA." *BMJ* 2012;345:e8343.

88: **trazodone is one of the most popular sleep aids in use today and may be useful in treating insomnia caused by SSRI antidepressants:** Saddichha, "Diagnosis and treatment of chronic insomnia."

88: **Overdosing on SADs is potentially lethal:** Saddichha, "Diagnosis and treatment of chronic insomnia."

89: **Suvorexant can also cause sleep paralysis:** Farkas R. (2013) "Suvorexant safety and efficacy." FDA Peripheral and Central Nervous System Drugs Advisory Committee. Available at: http://www.fda.gov.

89: **BDZs reduced sleep-onset time by 10 minutes and increased total sleep time by 32 minutes:** Buscemi N, Vandermeer B, Friesen C, et al. "The efficacy and safety of drug treatments for chronic insomnia in adults: a meta-analysis of RCTs." *J Gen Intern Med* 2007;22:1335–50.

89: **And suvorexant decreased sleep-onset time by a mere 2.3 minutes, with an increase in total sleep time of 21 minutes:** Kripke DF. "Is suvorexant a better choice than alternative hypnotics?" *F1000Research* 2015;4:456.

90: **a representative of the pharmaceutical industry commented, "If you forget how long you lay in bed tossing and turning, in some ways that's just as good as sleeping.":** Saul S. "Sleep drugs found only mildly effective, but wildly popular." *New York Times,* October 23, 2007. http://www.nytimes.com/2007/10/23/health/23drug.html.

91: **Long-term use of BDZs, Z-drugs, OTC sleep aids, and especially SADs results in tolerance:** Saddichha, "Diagnosis and treatment of chronic insomnia."

91: **Rebound insomnia can last from days to months, perpetuating dependence and addiction:** Saddichha, "Diagnosis and treatment of chronic insomnia."

91: **in reality, the two [Z-drugs and BDZs] are similar in terms of these adverse reactions:** Saddichha, "Diagnosis and treatment of chronic insomnia."

91: **These drugs [BDZs, SADs, and OTC sleep aids] have been linked to depression, dementia, and Alzheimer's disease, conditions also associated with impaired REM sleep:** Billioti de Gage S, Moride Y, Ducruet T, et al. "Benzodiazepine use and risk of Alzheimer's disease: case-control study." *BMJ* 2014;349:g5205. Lim AS, Kowgier M, Yu L, et al. "Sleep fragmentation and the risk of incident Alzheimer's disease and cognitive decline in older persons." *Sleep* 2013;36:1027–32.

92: **Even people taking fewer than eighteen pills per year had increased mortality:** Kripke DF, Langer RD, Kline LE. "Hypnotics' association with mortality or cancer: a matched cohort study." *BMJ Open* 2012;2:e000850.

92: **This is reinforced by the medicalization of sleep:** Lim, Kowgier, Yu, "Sleep fragmentation."

93: **Noise reduction is about identifying and managing the kinds of excessive stimulation that interfere with our innate tendency to sleep:** Naiman R. "Insomnia." In: Rakel D, ed. *Integrative medicine.* 3rd ed. (Philadelphia: Elsevier, 2015).

93: **A lack of adequate physical activity as well as chronic muscle tension, which is usually rooted in anxiety, are also examples of body noise:** Naiman, "Insomnia."

93: **Mindfulness-based stress reduction (MBSR) is a structured form of meditation that has been shown to be very useful in improving sleep:** Naiman, "Insomnia."

94: **CBT-I is particularly useful to mitigate excessive sleep effort:** Saddicha, "Diagnosis and treatment of chronic insomnia."

94: **Some botanical medicines and nutraceutical sleep supplements can help reduce insomnia:** Saddicha, "Diagnosis and treatment of chronic insomnia."

Chapter 7. Steroids

97: *Life* magazine, December 12, 1949.

97: **he continued to suffer severe flares that forced him to use crutches and finally a wheelchair:** Régnier C. "Hygeia versus Polymnia: Some French painters and their diseases." *Medicographia* 2005;27(3):279–87.

98: **Dufy accepted Homburger's offer and was admitted to Jewish Memorial Hospital in Boston in April 1950:** Homburger F, Bonner CD. "The treatment of Raoul Dufy's arthritis." *N Engl J Med* 1979;301(12): 669–73.

98: **Dr. Homburger noted that Dufy's response was "rapid, gratifying, and sustained":** Homburger, Bonner, "The treatment of Raoul Dufy's arthritis."

98: **Under anesthesia, more than 800 milliliters of pus were drained:** Homburger, Bonner, "The treatment of Raoul Dufy's arthritis."

98: **On March 12, 1953, Dufy wrote in his last letter to Dr. Homburger:** Mongan A. "Selections from the collection of Freddy and Regina T. Homburger; a loan exhibition, Harvard University, Fogg Art Museum [Cambridge, Mass.], April 2–24, 1971."

99: **Less than two weeks later, at the age of seventy-six, Raoul Dufy died:** Homburger, Bonner, "The treatment of Raoul Dufy's arthritis."

99: **As the most powerful anti-inflammatory agent yet discovered, cortisone transformed the practice of rheumatology almost overnight:** Le Fanu J. *The rise and fall of modern medicine.* Rev. ed. (New York: Basic Books, 2012).

99–100: **An estimated 1.2 percent of the US population over the age of twenty—more than 2.5 million people—received oral steroids between 1999 and 2008:** Overman RA, Yeh JY, Deal CL. "Prevalence of oral glucocorticoid usage in the United States: a general population perspective." *Arthritis Care Res* (Hoboken) 2013;65(2):294–8.

100: **The simple convenience of writing a prescription for a steroid has supplanted the traditional scientific method:** Le Fanu, *The rise and fall of modern medicine.*

102: **When initiating steroid treatment, experts agree on using the smallest dose for the shortest time:** Singh JA, Saag KG, Bridges SL, Jr., et al. 2015 "American College of Rheumatology guideline for the treatment of rheumatoid arthritis." *Arthritis Care Res* (Hoboken) 2015.

103: **In 1950, at the age of seventy-three, Raoul Dufy was the oldest patient ever to be treated with cortisone:** Homburger, Bonner, "The treatment of Raoul Dufy's arthritis."

104: **Between 1997 and 2014, the FDA received reports of ninety serious neurologic events, some fatal, related to epidural injection of steroids:** Racoosin JA, Seymour SM, Cascio L, Gill R. "Serious neurologic events after epidural glucocorticoid injection: the FDA's risk assessment." *N Engl J Med* 2015;373(24):2299–301.

Chapter 8. Nonsteroidal Anti-Inflammatory Drugs (NSAIDs)

110: **Currently, there are at least twenty prescription-only formulations, as well as a multitude of brand-name and generic versions of OTC NSAIDs:** *Consumer Reports.* "The nonsteroidal anti-inflammatory drugs: treating osteoarthritis and pain: comparing effectiveness, safety, and price." July 2013.

116: **Improved diet and exercise can lead to weight loss, and weight loss often reduces chronic pain:** Narouze S, Souzdalnitski D. "Obesity and chronic pain: systematic review of prevalence and implications for pain practice." *Reg Anesth Pain Med* 2015;40:91–111.

117: **Except for fish, eggs, and high-quality dairy products, animal foods are minimized:** Minihane AM,

Vinoy S, Russell WR, et al. "Low-grade inflammation, diet composition and health: current research evidence and its translation." *Br J Nutr* 2015;114:999–1012.

117: **it is well established that improved sleep can result in decreased chronic pain:** Passos GS, Pyares D, Santana M, et al. "Exercise improves immune function, antidepressive response, and sleep quality in patients with chronic primary insomnia." *BioMed Res Internat* 2014:Article 498961, 7p.

117: **Smoking is associated with increased chronic pain:** Petre B, Torbey S, Griffith JW, et al. "Smoking increases risk of pain chronification through shared corticostriatal circuitry." *Hum Brain Map* 2015;36:683–94.

117: **It [arnica] has also been shown to decrease pain and swelling after surgery:** Brinkhaus B, Wilkens JM, Ludtke R, et al. "Homeopathic arnica therapy in patients receiving knee surgery: results of three randomised double-blind trials." *Compl Ther Med* 2006;14:237–46.

117: **Additionally, arnica has been shown to decrease pain associated with mild to moderate osteoarthritis:** Widrig R, Suter A, Saller R, et al. "Choosing between NSAID and arnica for topical treatment of hand osteoarthritis in a randomized double-blind study." *Rheumatol Internat* 2007;27:585–91.

118: **curcumin supplementation has been found to be as effective as ibuprofen for osteoarthritis of the knee:** Kuptniratsaikul V, Daipratham P, Taechaarpornkul W, et al. "Efficacy and safety of *Curcuma domestica* extracts compared with ibuprofen in patients with knee osteoarthritis: a multicenter study." *Clin Interv Aging* 2014;9: 451–58.

118: **Extracts of a familiar relative of turmeric — ginger — have been shown to modestly improve pain associated with osteoarthritis of the knee:** Altman RD, Marcussen KC. "Effects of a ginger extract on knee pain in patients with osteoarthritis." *Arthrit Rheumatol* 2001;44:2531–538.

118: **Acupuncture can also work as an alternative to chronic NSAID use:** Vickers A, Phil D, Cronin A, et al. "Acupuncture for chronic pain: individual patient data meta-analysis." *Arch Intern Med* 2012;172:1444–53.

118: **Mind-body approaches, such as hypnosis, guided imagery, and guided meditation, can provide relief by teaching patients to change their perception of painful sensations:** Astin JA. "Mind-body therapies for the management of pain." *Clin J Pain* 2004;20:27–32.

Chapter 9. Psychiatric Medications for Adults

123: **Adverse reactions to drugs are the fourth leading cause of death in our country:** Institute of Medicine (IOM). "To err is human: building a safer health system." Washington, DC: National Academy Press, 2000. Lazarou J, Pomeranz BH, Corey PN. "Incidence of adverse drug reactions in hospitalized patients. A meta-analysis of prospective studies." *JAMA* 1998;279:1200–1205. Gurwitz JH, Field TS, Avorn J, et al. "Incidence and preventability of adverse drug events in nursing homes." *Am J Med* 2000;109:87–94.

124: **In 2010, antidepressants were the second most commonly prescribed medications:** National Institute of

Mental Health (NIMH). Director's Blog: "Antidepressants: a complicated picture." December 6, 2011. http://www.nimh.nih.gov/about/director/2011/antidepressants-a-complicated-picture.shtml.

124: **The rate of antidepressant use across all age groups exploded from 1988 to 2008, increasing nearly 400 percent:** Pratt L, Brody DJ, Gu Q. "Antidepressant Use in Persons Aged 12 and Over: United States, 2005–2008." *NCHS Data Brief. No 76.* October 2011. Centers for Disease Control and Prevention (CDC). *NCHS Data Brief No. 76,* October 2011. http://www.cdc.gov/nchs/data/databriefs/db76.htm. National Center for Health Statistics (NCHS). "Health, United States, 2010: with special feature on death and dying." Table 95. Hyattsville, MD, 2011.

124: **One study showed that medical professionals other than psychiatrists write 80 percent of antidepressant prescriptions:** Mark T, Levit K, Buck J. "Datapoints: psychotropic drug prescriptions by medical specialty." *Psychiatry Svc* 2009;60:1167.

125: **Use by pregnant women may increase the risk of autism in their children, as well as birth defects:** Bérard A, Iessa N, Chaabane S, et al. "The risk of major cardiac malformations associated with paroxetine use during the first trimester of pregnancy: a systematic review and meta-analysis." *Br J Clin Pharmacol* 2016. doi: 10.1111/bcp.12849.

125: **Although they have a better side-effect profile, the efficacy of SGAs is not as good as that of the first-generation drugs:** Leucht S, Corves C, Arbter D, et al. "Second-generation versus first-generation antipsychotic drugs for schizophrenia: a meta-analysis." *Lancet* 2009;373:31–41.

125: **In 2013, Abilify was the number one prescribed psychotropic medication and the overall top drug by sales:** Brooks, M. "Top 100 selling drugs of 2013." *Medscape,* January 30, 2014. http://www.medscape.com/viewarticle/820011.

125: **Between 2001 and 2011, the US Veterans Health Administration and Department of Defense spent almost $850 million on Seroquel:** "VA/Defense mental health drug expenditures since 2001. May 2012 drug totals." http://cdn.govexec.com/media/gbc/docs/pdfs_edit/051712bb1_may2012drugtotals.pdf.

126: **Furthermore, physicians prescribe these medications off label for insomnia, anxiety, stress, and mild mood disorders:** Alexander GC, Gallagher SA, Mascola A, et al: "Increasing off-label use of antipsychotic medications in the United States, 1995–2008." *Pharmacoepidemiol Drug Saf* 2011;20:177–84.

126: **More importantly, long-term use of antipsychotic medication does not provide more benefits than short-term use:** Wunderink L, Nieboer RM, Wiersma D, et al. "Recovery in remitted first-episode psychosis at 7 years of follow-up of an early dose reduction/discontinuation or maintenance treatment strategy: long-term follow-up of a 2-year randomized clinical trial." *JAMA Psychiatry* 2013; 70:913–20.

126: **Together, they [anxiety disorders] cost the United States more than $42 billion a year:** Anxiety and Depression

Association of America (ADAA). "Facts and statistics." Last updated September 2014. http://www.adaa.org/about-adaa/press-room/facts-statistics.

127: **A 2013 survey showed that Xanax has consistently been the number one prescribed psychiatric medication, with Ativan at number five and Valium in eleventh place:** Grohol J. "Top 25 psychiatric medication prescriptions for 2013." *Psych Central.* http://psychcentral.com/lib/top-25-psychiatric-medication-prescriptions-for-2013/.

130–31: **Many options are available for managing depression and anxiety without drugs:** Weil A. *Spontaneous Happiness* (New York: Little, Brown, 2011).

131: **There is good scientific evidence, for example, for the antidepressant effects of exercise:** Archer T, Josefsson T, Lindwall M. "Effects of physical exercise on depressive symptoms and biomarkers in depression." *CNS Neurol Disord Targets* 2014;13:1640–53.

131: **and supplemental fish oil:** Grosso G, Galvano F, Marventano S, et al. "Omega-3 fatty acids and depression: scientific evidence and biological mechanisms." *Oxid Med Cell Longev* 2014; 2014: 313570. doi: 10.1155/2014/313570.

Chapter 10. Psychiatric Medications for Children and Adolescents

135: **The costs add up to more than $240 billion in annual spending to cover health care, educational services, and decreased productivity:** Perou R, Bitsko RH, Blumberg SJ, et al. "Mental health surveillance among children—United States, 2005–2011." *MMWR* 2013;62 (suppl 2):1–35.

135: **According to the US National Health and Nutrition Examination Survey, 6 percent of US teens reported using a psychiatric medication in the past month:** Jonas B, Gu Q, Albertorio-Diaz JR. "Psychotropic medication use among adolescents: United States, 2005–2010." *NCHS data brief no. 135*, December 2013. http://www.cdc.gov/nchs/data/databriefs/db135.pdf.

135: **A 2014 report from the Agency for Healthcare Research and Quality:** Agency for Healthcare Research and Quality (AHRQ). *Medical expenditure panel survey, 2014.* http://meps.ahrq.gov/mepsweb/data_files/publications/st434/stat434.pdf.

137: **In depressed children twelve or younger, antidepressants were found to be less effective than in adolescents:** Bridge JA, Iyengar S, Salary CB, et al. "Clinical response and risk for reported suicidal ideation and suicide attempts in pediatric antidepressant treatment: a meta-analysis of randomized controlled trials." *JAMA* 2007;297:1683–96.

138: **Also, these rats [rats treated with Prozac before maturity] show problems with sexual behavior as adults:** Iñiguez SD, Alcantara LF, Warren BL, et al. "Fluoxetine exposure during adolescence alters responses to aversive stimuli in adulthood." *J Neurosci* 2014;34:1007–21.

138–39: **A study of children diagnosed with bipolar disorder found that about 60 percent had been treated previously** with an antidepressant or a stimulant medication: Cicero D, Rif S, El-Maliakh et al. "Antidepressant exposure in bipolar children." *Psychiatry* 2003;66:317–22.

140: **the majority of SGAs are prescribed off label for depression, anxiety, insomnia, and disruptive behavior— without much being known about their long-term risks versus benefits:** Rettew DC, Greenblatt J, Kamon J, et al. "Antipsychotic Medication Prescribing in Children Enrolled in Medicaid." *Pediatrics* 2015;135:658–65.

140: **Only a small percentage of children and teens who are prescribed these powerful drugs also receive psychotherapy:** Olfson M, King M, Schoenbaum M. "Treatment of young people with antipsychotic medications in the United States." *JAMA Psychiatry* 2015;72:867–74.

140: **Some studies even suggest a reduction in brain volume over time with the use of these medications:** Ho B-C, Andreasen NC, Ziebell S, et al. "Long-term antipsychotic treatment and brain volumes: a longitudinal study of first-episode schizophrenia." *Arch Gen Psychiatry* 2011;68:128–37.

140–41: **in one study, Abilify use resulted in a weight gain of 10 pounds after eleven weeks; Zyprexa, 19 pounds; Seroquel, 13 pounds; and Risperdal, 12 pounds:** Correll CU, Manu P, Olshanskiy V, et al. "Cardiometabolic risk of second-generation antipsychotic medications during first-time use in children and adolescents." *JAMA* 2009;302:1765–73.

142: **In one study, teens prescribed benzodiazepines were ten times more likely to misuse these medications to**

get high: Boyd CJ, Austic E, Epstein-Ngo Q, et al. "A prospective study of adolescents' nonmedical use of anxiolytic and sleep medication." *Psychol Addict Behav* 2015;29:184–91.

143–44: **A diet of unprocessed whole foods...limits inflammation in the body and promotes better mental health:** Jacka FN, Kremer PJ, Berk M, et al. "A prospective study of diet quality and mental health in adolescents." *PloS One* 2011;6:e24805.

144: **Recent research links depression with increased inflammation:** Miller AH and Raison CL. "The role of inflammation in depression: from evolutionary imperative to modern treatment target." *Nature Rev Immunol* 2016: 16, 22–34; doi: 10.1038/nri.2015.5.

Chapter 11. Medications for Attention Deficit Hyperactivity Disorder (ADHD)

149: **according to the latest government statistics, about 4.2 million of them [children] are taking a psychostimulant medication:** Centers for Disease Control and Prevention (CDC). "New data: Medication and behavior treatment." Last updated March 15, 2015. http://www.cdc.gov/ncbddd/adhd/data.html.

150: **In 2010, a researcher showed that children born in August were more than twice as likely to be diagnosed with ADHD:** Elder T. "The importance of relative standards in ADHD diagnoses: Evidence based on exact birth dates." *J Health Econ* 2010;29:641–56.

150: **Another study, described in the book *The ADHD Explosion:*** Hinshaw S, Sheffler R. *The ADHD Explosion: myths, medication, money, and today's push for performance* (Oxford: Oxford University Press, 2014).

150–51: **in 2011 the ADHD rate in Indiana was 13.8 percent, almost double that of neighboring Illinois:** Centers for Disease Control and Prevention (CDC). "New data: medication and behavior treatment." Last updated March 15, 2015. http://www.cdc.gov/ncbddd/adhd/data.html.

151: **One study showed that of children who were rated by one teacher as having inattention symptoms of ADHD, fewer than 50 percent were so rated by their teacher in the following year:** Rabiner DL, Murray DW, Rosen L, et al. "Instability in teacher ratings of children's inattentive symptoms: implications for the assessment of ADHD." *J Dev Behav Pediatr* 2010;31:175–80.

152: **The cost of ADHD drugs ranges from $15 to $500 a month.** Brody B. "The shocking cost of your child's ADHD." *Fiscal Times,* April 1, 2013.

152: **Even though children are still the primary users, in recent years the greatest increase in expenditure on them has been among adults.** *Express Scripts Report.* "Turning attention to ADHD: US medication trends for attention deficit hyperactivity disorder." March 2014.

153: **A recent study showed that 62 percent of children of parents with a history of major depression, bipolar disorder, or schizophrenia developed psychotic symptoms while taking psychostimulants:** Mackenzie

L, Abidi S, Fisher HL, et al. "Stimulant medication and psychotic symptoms in offspring of children with mental illness." *Pediatrics* 2016;137:1–10.

153: **The most famous of these was the so-called Multi-modal Treatment of Attention Deficit Hyperactivity Disorder (MTA) study:** Jensen PS, Arnold LE, Swanson JM, et al. "3-year follow-up of the NIMH MTA study." *J Am Acad Child Adolesc Psychiatry* 2007;46: 989–1002.

153–54: **"The modest significant advantages we found at the twenty-four-month assessment for the MTA Medication Algorithm...were completely lost by thirty-six months":** Jensen et al., "3-year follow-up of the NIMH MTA study."

154: **Results of another long-term investigation, the Preschool Attention Deficit Hyperactivity Treatment Study:** Riddle MA, Yershova K, Lazzaretto D, et al. "The Preschool Attention-Deficit/Hyperactivity Disorder Treatment Study (PATS) 6-year follow-up." *J Am Acad Child Adolesc Psychiatry* 2013;52:264–78.

154: **One study measured the thickness of the cerebral cortex in the frontal lobe of the brain as children grew:** Shaw P, Malek M, Watson B, et al. "Trajectories of cerebral cortical development in childhood and adolescence and adult attention-deficit/hyperactivity disorder." *Biol Psychiatry* 2013;74:599–606.

155: **The long-term studies that could give us answers are hard to do with children, but they have been done**

with rats, and the results should give us pause: Marco E, Adriani W, Ruocco LA, et al. "Neurobehavioral adaptations to methylphenidate: the issue of early adolescent exposure." *Neurosci Biobehav Rev* 2011;35:1722–39.

155: **The conclusions…highlighted the "urgent need for large randomized controlled trials of non-pharmacological treatments":** Storebø OJ, Ramstad E, Krogh HB, et al. "Methylphenidate for children and adolescents with attention deficit hyperactivity disorder." *Cochrane Database Syst Rev* 2015 Nov 25;11:CD009885.

155–56: **In one survey, nearly two-thirds of students at a large mid-Atlantic university had been offered stimulant medication, and 31 percent admitted to abusing ADHD drugs:** Watson GLF, Arcona AP, Anotonuccio DO. "The ADHD drug abuse crisis on American college campuses" *Ethical Hum Psychol Psychiatry* 2015;17:1–16.

156: **As quoted in one study, a young college student said, "You swallow Adderall to study and snort it for fun":** Varga MD. "Adderall abuse on college campuses: a comprehensive literature review." *J Evid Based Soc Work* 2012;9:293–313.

156: **a 2011 study published in the prestigious British medical journal the *Lancet* showed that 64 percent of children improved significantly when placed on an elimination diet:** Pelsser LM, Frankena K, Toorman J, et al., "Effects of a restricted elimination diet on the behaviour of children with attention-deficit hyperactivity disorder (INCA study): a randomised controlled trial." *Lancet* 2011;377:494–503.

157: **Omega-3 fatty acids, found primarily in fish, are generally deficient in affected children; supplementation with fish oil can be beneficial:** Bloch M, Qawasmi A. "Omega-3 fatty acid supplementation for the treatment of children with attention-deficit/hyperactivity disorder symptomatology: systematic review and meta-analysis." *J Am Acad Child Adolesc Psychiatry* 2011;50:991–1000.

157: **one study did find that giving supplemental probiotics to infants significantly decreased their chances of developing ADHD:** Pärtty A, Kalliomäki M, Wacklin P, et al. "A possible link between early probiotic intervention and the risk of neuropsychiatric disorders later in childhood: a randomized trial." *Pediatr Res* 2015;77: 823–28.

Chapter 12. Opioids and the Treatment of Chronic Pain

159: **in 2010 American physicians prescribed enough [opioids] to treat every adult in the country around the clock for a month:** Centers for Disease Control and Prevention (CDC). "Prescription painkiller overdoses in the US." http://www.cdc.gov/vitalsigns/PainkillerOverdoses/ index.html. Last updated November 1, 2011.

162: **for more than 1.5 billion people worldwide and more than 100 million Americans, the problem lasts more than several months, becoming chronic:** IOM (Institute of Medicine). *Relieving pain in America: a blueprint for transforming prevention, care, education, and research.* (Washington, DC: The National Academies Press, 2011).

162: **Involvement of these other brain regions appears to be related to difficult symptoms that often accompany chronic pain:** Tsang A, Von Korff M, Lee S, et al. "Common chronic pain conditions in developed and developing countries: Gender and age differences and comorbidity with depression-anxiety disorders." *J Pain* 2008;9:883–91. Smallwood RF, Laird AR, Ramage AE, et al. "Structural brain anomalies and chronic pain: a quantitative meta-analysis of gray matter volume." *J Pain* 2013;14:663–75.

164: **"It is remarkable that opioid treatment of long-term/ chronic non-cancer pain does not seem to fulfill any of the key outcome opioid treatment goals.":** Eriksen J, Sjøgren P, Bruera E, et al. "Critical issues on opioids in chronic non-cancer pain: an epidemiological study." *Pain* 2006;125:172–79.

166: **This followed a call by noted pain clinicians to not undertreat pain:** Apkarian AV, Baliki MN, Farmer MA. "Predicting transition to chronic pain." *Curr Opin Neurol* 2013;26:360–7.

166: **Overall, opioid prescriptions have quadrupled since 1999, with a similar sharp increase in opioid-related overdoses, injuries, and deaths:** Deyo RA, Mirza SK, Turner JA, et al. "Overtreating chronic back pain: time to back off?" *J Am Board Fam Med* 2009;22:62–8.

166: **Prescription opioid abuse and misuse cost the United States more than $60 billion each year:** Gusovsky D. "America's painkiller epidemic grips the workplace." CNBC. December 15, 2015. http://www.cnbc.com/

2015/12/15/80-percent-of-workplaces-face-this-drug
-scourge.html.

167: **Dr. Richard A. Friedman...wrote in a *New York Times* editorial in 2015:** PBS. "The opium kings: opium throughout history." Frontline. Accessed February 11, 2015 at http://www.pbs.org/wgbh/pages/frontline/shows/heroin/etc/history.html.

167: **By 2011, many of the clinicians involved in promoting increased opioid use were publicly acknowledging that there were significant problems:** Catan T, Perez E. "A pain drug champion has second thoughts." *Wall Street Journal,* December 11, 2011. http://online.wsj.com/news/articles/SB1000142412788732447830457817334265704604.

168: **A recent review of more than twenty lower-back-pain studies:** Kizhakkeveettil A, Rose K, Kadar GE. "Integrative therapies for low back pain that include complementary and alternative medicine care—a systematic review." *Glob Adv Health Med.* 2014;3(5):49–64.

168: **the Oregon Pain Management Commission's integrative initiative:** The Oregon Pain Management Commission (OPMC). http://www.oregon.gov/oha/OHPR/PMC/pages/index.aspx.

Chapter 13. Antihypertensive Drugs

174: **In 2014, 32.5 percent of American adults had a diagnosis of high blood pressure:** National Center for Health Statistics (NCHS), "Health, United States, 2014: with special feature on adults aged 55–64." Hyattsville, MD, 2015.

175: **Research continues to indicate that careful blood pressure control markedly decreases risk:** Siu, AL. "Screening for high blood pressure in adults: US Preventive Services Task Force recommendation statement." *Ann Intern Med.* 2015;163(10):778–86.

176: **Recent research findings suggest that it is desirable to lower pressures that are even slightly above the 120/80 previously considered normal:** Sundstrom J, Arima H, Jackson R, Turnbull F, RahimiK, Chalmers J, Woodward M, Neal B. "Effects of blood pressure reduction in mild hypertension: a systematic review and meta-analysis." *Ann Intern Med.* 2015;162:184–91.

176: **In 2010, the United States spent nearly $42.9 billion on the management of hypertension:** Davis K. "Expenditures for hypertension among adults age 18 and older, 2010: estimates for the UW civilian noninstitutionalized population." *Statistical brief no. 404.* April 2013. Agency for Healthcare Research and Quality (AHRQ). http://www.meps.ahrq.gov/mepsweb/data_files/publications/st404/stat404.shtml.

178: **Recent studies indicate that beta blockers are probably *not* the best first choice for blood pressure management in most people:** Farooq U. "2014 guideline for the management of high blood pressure (Eighth Joint National Committee): take-home messages." *Med Clin N Am.* 2015;99:733–8.

182: **There are any number of ways to treat—and prevent—high blood pressure:** Plotnikoff GA, Dusek J. "Hypertension." In Rakel D, ed. *Integrative medicine.* 3rd ed. (Philadelphia: Elsevier, 2010).

182: **And several recent studies indicate that eating unsalted nuts can lower blood pressure:** Mohammadifard N, Salehi-Abargouei A, Salas-Salvado J, Guasch-Ferre M, Humphries K, Sarrafzadegan N. "The effect of tree nut, peanut, and soy nut consumption on blood pressure: a systematic review and meta-analysis of randomized controlled clinical trials." *Am J Clin Nutr.* 2015; 101(5):966–82.

183: **A 2013 review found that reducing sodium from between 9 and 12 grams daily to between 5 and 6 grams daily has a significant beneficial effect:** Aburto NJ, Ziolkovska A, et al., "Effect of lower sodium intake on health: systematic review and meta-analyses." *BMJ* 2013:346:f1326.

183: **A number of lifestyle factors favorably influence blood pressure:** Oza R, Barcellano M. "Nonpharmacologic management of hypertension: what works?" *Am Fam Physician.* 2015;91(11):772–6.

183: **Yoga shows promise in what little research we have so far:** Posadzki P, Cramer H, Kuzdzal A, Lee MS, Ernst E. "Yoga for hypertension: a systematic review of randomized clinical trials." *Complement Ther Med.* 2014;22(3): 511–22.

183: **as does tai chi:** Hartley L, Flowers N, Lee MS, Ernst E, Rees K. "Tai chi for primary prevention of cardiovascular disease." *Cochrane Database Syst Rev.* 2014;9;4:CD010366. doi: 10.1002/14651858.CD010366.pub2.

183: **Relaxation training, such as breathing exercises, meditation, and biofeedback, lowers blood pressure:** Plotnikoff, "Hypertension."

184: **Research indicates that people who are less isolated and more connected with others are less likely to be hypertensive:** Yang YC, Boen C, Mullan HK. "Social relationships and hypertension in late life: evidence from a nationally representative longitudinal study of older adults." *J Aging Health.* 2015;27(3):403–31.

184: **A number of supplements have shown promise in lowering blood pressure:** "Natural medicines in the clinical management of hypertension." http://naturaldatabase .therapeuticresearch.com.

Chapter 14. Medications for Diabetes

187: **The cost of diabetes in 2007 was estimated at $174 billion and growing:** American Diabetes Association (ADA). "Economic costs of diabetes in the U.S. in 2007." *Diabetes Care* 2008;31:596–615.

187: **Treatment plans are provided to doctors, nurses, and other health professionals to help optimize care:** Garber AJ, et al. "AACE/ACE comprehensive diabetes management algorithm 2015." *Endocr Practice* 2015;21: 438–47.

190: **A 2007 summary of the known science on the safety of rosiglitazone stunned the medical community:** Nissen SE, Wolski K. "Effect of rosiglitazone on the risk of myocardial infarction and death from cardiovascular causes." *N Engl J Med* 2007;356:2457–71.

Chapter 15. Medications for Osteopenia and Other Preconditions

197: **Based on this definition, more than half of women and a third of men over age fifty in the United States are believed to have osteopenia:** Looker AC, Melton LJ, et al. "Prevalence and trends in low femur bone density among older US adults: NHANES 2005–2006 compared with NHANES III." *J Bone Miner Res* 2010;25: 64–71.

199: **Today the drugs [bisphosphonates] are also given to children with inherited skeletal disorders, such as osteogenesis imperfecta:** Francis MD, Valent DJ. "Historical perspectives on the clinical development of bisphosphonates in the treatment of bone diseases." *J Musculoskelet Neuronal Interact* 2007;7:2–8.

199: **Decades of research have shown the bisphosphonates act in the body as anti-resorptive agents:** Rodan GA, Fleisch HA. "Bisphosphonates: mechanisms of action." *J Clin Invest* 1996;97:2692–96.

200: **Among the many adverse reactions to [bisphosphonates] are atypical fractures of the thigh bones:** Odvina CV, Zerwekh JE, et al. "Severely suppressed bone turnover: a potential complication of alendronate therapy." *J Clin Endocrinol Metab* 2005;90:1294–1301.

201: **osteonecrosis of the jaw:** Khosla S, Burr D, et al. "Bisphosphonate-associated osteonecrosis of the jaw: report of a task force of the American Society for Bone and Mineral Research." *J Bone Miner Res* 2007;22:1479–91.

201: **the number of osteoporotic patients needed to receive treatment for three years to prevent one hip fracture is forty-five for vitamin D, forty-eight for strontium ranelate, and ninety-one for bisphosphonates:** Sweet MG, Sweet JM, et al. "Diagnosis and treatment of osteoporosis." *Am Fam Physician* 2009;79:193–200.

201–2: **For managing the precondition osteopenia with bisphosphonates, the number needed to treat is very high, meaning the drugs are not very effective:** Ringe JD, Doherty JG. "Absolute risk reduction in osteoporosis: assessing treatment efficacy by number needed to treat." *Rheumatol Int* 2010;30:863–869. Eriksen EF. "Treatment of osteopenia." *Rev Endocr and Metab Disord* 2012;13:209–23.

202: **When hormones are advised, the transdermal application of bioidentical products (those with the same chemical structures as the body's own hormones) may cause fewer side effects and have a somewhat lower risk profile than other forms of estrogen:** Holtorf K. "The bioidentical hormone debate: are bioidentical hormones (estradiol, estriol, and progesterone) safer or more efficacious than commonly used synthetic versions in hormone replacement therapy?" *Postgrad Med* 2009;121: 73–85.

203: **Research indicates that the trace element strontium stimulates bone formation and is effective for preventing bone loss:** Reginster JY, Deroisy R, et al. "Prevention of early postmenopausal bone loss by strontium ranelate: the randomized, two-year-double-masked, dose-ranging, placebo-controlled PREVOS trial." *Osteoporos Int* 2002; 13:925–31.

204: **Research shows that weight-bearing exercises like walking are effective for increasing bone density of the hips and spine:** Iwamoto J, Sato Y, et al. "Effectiveness of exercise in the treatment of lumbar spinal stenosis, knee osteoarthritis, and osteoporosis," *Aging Clin Exp Res* 2010;2:116–22.

205: **Research shows that diet and exercise are twice as effective as the drug metformin (Glucophage, Glumetza) for reducing the progression of pre-diabetes to diabetes:** Knowler WC, Barrett-Connor E, et al. "Reduction in the incidence of type 2 diabetes with lifestyle intervention or metformin." *New Engl J Med* 2002;346:393–403.

Chapter 16. Overmedication of Children

207: **An estimated 263.6 million prescriptions were written for children and adolescents in the United States in 2010**: Chai G, Governale L, McMahon AW, et al. "Trends of outpatient prescription drug utilization in US children, 2002–2010." *Pediatr* 2012;130(1):23–31.

208: **studies show that use [of OTC cough and cold medicines] in the two- to six-year-old age group has actually increased:** Mazer-Amirshahi M, Rasooly I, Brooks G, et al. "The impact of pediatric labeling changes on prescribing patterns of cough and cold medications." *Pediatr* 2014;165(5):1024–8.e1.

208: **Nonetheless, the 2012 annual report of the American Association of Poison Control Centers lists OTC cough-cold medications among the top three products associated with fatality in children under age five:** Mowry JB, Spyker DA, Cantilena LR Jr, et al. "2012 Annual Report of the American Association of Poison Control Centers' National Poison Data System (NPDS): 30th Annual Report." *Clin Toxicol (Phila)* 2013;51(10): 949–1229.

209: **guaifenesin is ineffective; large randomized studies have shown it to have no measurable effect:** Hoffer-Schaefer A, Rozycki HJ, Yopp MA, et al. "Guaifenesin has no effect on sputum volume or sputum properties in adolescents and adults with acute respiratory tract infections." *Respir Care* 2014;59(5):631–6.

209: **Phenylephrine also lacks demonstrated effectiveness, and there are no studies of its safety in children:** Hatton RC, Winterstein AG, McKelvey RP, et al. "Efficacy and safety of oral phenylephrine: systematic review and meta-analysis." *Ann Pharmacother.* 2007;41(3):381–90.

209: **AAP clinical policy statements dating from 1997 have found no studies to support the safety or efficacy of dextromethorphan in pediatrics and no indications for its use:** American Academy of Pediatrics (AAP). Committee on Drugs. "Use of codeine- and dextromethorphan-containing cough remedies in children." *Pediatr* 1997;99(6):918–20.

209: **According to the 2007 National Health Interview Survey, an estimated 2.9 million children and ado-**

lescents use some type of dietary supplement: Wu CH, Wang CC, Kennedy J. "The prevalence of herb and dietary supplement use among children and adolescents in the United States: results from the 2007 National Health Interview Survey." *Complement Ther Med* 2013;21(4): 358–63.

210: **Buckwheat (dark) honey, in those over one year of age for reducing nighttime cough:** Oduwole O, Meremikwu MM, Oyo-Ita A, et al. "Honey for acute cough in children." *Cochrane Database Syst Rev* 2014;12: CD007094.

210: **Use of oral zinc in liquid or lozenge form is associated with fewer colds in children:** Fashner J, Ericson K, Werner S. "Treatment of the common cold in children and adults." *Am Fam Physician* 2012;86(2):153–9.

211: **A 2011 AAP statement cautioned that children and adolescents should not consume energy drinks:** Committee on Nutrition and the Council on Sports Medicine and Fitness. "Sports drinks and energy drinks for children and adolescents: are they appropriate?" *Pediatr* 127(6):1182–9.

212: **Insufficient sleep has been linked to overweight and obesity in children and may be treated with prescription or OTC medications:** Gurnani M, Birken C, Hamilton J. "Childhood obesity: causes, consequences, and management." *Pediatr Clin North Am* 2015;62(4):821–40.

213: **In adults, long-term treatment with metformin has been shown to increase the risk of vitamin B_{12} deficiency:** Gurnani, "Childhood obesity."

213: **We have very limited data on the impact of statins in children:** Gurnani, "Childhood obesity."

214: **Long-term studies on its [orlistat's] effects in children and adolescents are lacking:** Gurnani, "Childhood obesity."

214: **surgery...should be reserved for carefully screened, dangerously obese adolescents:** Inge TH, Courcoulas AP, Jenkins TM, et al. "Weight Loss and Health Status 3 Years after Bariatric Surgery in Adolescents." *N Engl J Med* 2016 ;374(2):113–23.

Chapter 17. Overmedication of the Elderly

220: **These OTC remedies [for sleep] are particularly attractive to older people, many of whom find good sleep elusive:** McCall, WV. "Sleep in the elderly: burden, diagnosis, and treatment." *Prim Care Companion J Clin Psychiatry* 2004;6(1).

221: **Studies of older hip fracture patients have shown that 16 to 62 percent develop delirium:** Kyziridis T. "Postoperative delirium after hip fracture treatment—a review of the current literature." *Psychosoc Med.* 2006;3: Doc01 (PMC2736510).

221: **Moreover, benzodiazepines also increase the risk of falls and can even precipitate delirium by making people groggy and confused:** Sithamparanathan, K, Sadera, L, Leung, L. "Adverse effects of benzodiazepine use in elderly people: a meta-analysis." *Asian J Gerontol Geriatr* 2012;7(2):107–11.

221: **The American Geriatrics Society felt so strongly about avoiding benzodiazepine use in the elderly:** American Geriatrics Society. "Ten things physicians and patients should question." Choosing Wisely by ABIM. Released February 21, 2013 (1–5), and February 27, 2014 (6–10); Revised April 23, 2015 (2, 3, 6, 7, 8, and 10). http://www .choosingwisely.org/societies/american-geriatrics-society/.

222: **long-term suppression of it [stomach acid] with drugs like omeprazole can have serious consequences:** McDonald EG, Milligan J, Frenette C, Lee TC. "Continuous proton pump inhibitor therapy and the associated risk of recurrent *Clostridium difficile* infection." *JAMA Intern Med.* 2015;175(5):784–91.

222: **tricyclic antidepressants, like their antihistamine relatives, can cause urinary obstruction and constipation as well as increase the risk of falls and delirium:** American Geriatrics Society. "American Geriatrics Society 2015 Updated Beers Criteria for Potentially Inappropriate Medication Use in Older Adults." *J Am Geriatr Soc* 2015;63(11):22227–46.

223: **Among those over the age of sixty-five, the incidence of polypharmacy, defined as being on five or more medications at one time, rose from 30.6 percent to 35.8 percent from 2005 to 2011:** Qato DM, Wilder J, Schumm LP, et al. "Changes in prescription and over-the-counter medication and dietary supplement use among older adults in the United States, 2005 vs 2011." *JAMA Intern Med* 2016;176:473–82.

About the Author

ANDREW WEIL, MD, is the author of fourteen previous books, including *Spontaneous Healing, 8 Weeks to Optimum Health, Healthy Aging,* and *Spontaneous Happiness.* A graduate of Harvard College and Harvard Medical School, he is professor of public health, clinical professor of medicine, and the Lovell-Jones Professor of Integrative Rheumatology at the University of Arizona, as well as director of the University of Arizona Center for Integrative Medicine.

Dr. Weil is the editorial director of DrWeil.com, the leading online resource for healthy living based on the philosophy of integrative medicine. He authors the popular "Self-Healing" newsletter and columns for *Prevention* magazine and is a frequent guest on numerous national talk shows. He lives in Arizona.